# CURING
# STUBBORN
# DEPRESSION

## EMERGING & BREAKTHROUGH THERAPIES
## FOR TREATMENT-RESISTANT DEPRESSION

## PAUL B. FITZGERALD, PhD, MBBS

Hatherleigh Press is committed to preserving and protecting the natural resources of the earth. Environmentally responsible and sustainable practices are embraced within the company's mission statement.

Visit us at www.hatherleighpress.com.

# CURING STUBBORN DEPRESSION

Library of Congress Cataloging-in-Publication Data is available.

ISBN: 978-1-57826-937-2

Cover by Carolyn Kasper

Printed in the United States

10 9 8 7 6 5 4 3 2 1

# CONTENTS

# INTRODUCTION

I N THE LAST decade or two, many millions of words have been written about depression, in the accounts of those who have lived through it, in textbooks, in research studies, and in self-help books. It is a condition which is now widely discussed in newspapers, on television and in social media. It is also a disorder around which opinions have always been, and remain, frequently polarized. Is depression a psychological condition? Is it a medical disorder? Is it a condition of modern society: resulting from a breakdown in family and societal relationships, from a loss of meaning and self-worth associated with traditional roles? Is depression a disorder of society or of individuals? Is depression a single clinical entity or a label used to describe many different experiences? How much of what we call depression has been a successful attempt by psychiatrists and the pharmaceutical industry to medicalize aspects of the normal human experience?

The purpose of this book is not to re-prosecute these arguments. The depression that will be discussed is profoundly a clinical disorder. By that I mean it is a condition that results in patients presenting to clinicians: be they family physicians, psychologists, or psychiatrists, with markedly disabling symptoms and impaired quality of life. Patients in the throes of clinical depression are not usually interested in profound philosophical discussions as to the nature of experience or of the role of mental health treatment in society. They are suffering, just as patients suffer with other mental health and physical conditions and seek pathways out of this suffering. How their depression has arisen, whether through a psychological trauma, social disengagement, or derangement of some element of the neurobiology of their brain function, may have some relevance in determining how they should be treated, but at an individual level. Patients may be interested in what has caused their depression but typically this is not a profoundly philosophical consideration. They want to know why they have become ill and more importantly how do they get better, and usually how to do the latter as quickly as possible.

Getting better is usually the challenge. Over recent decades, many countries, but undisputedly not all, have done a very good job at reducing the stigma associated with depression and other mental health conditions. There have been concerted public health efforts to address this stigma, often interacting with the willingness of public figures—usually politicians and sportspeople—to come forward and discuss their struggles. In some places, these efforts have occurred alongside specific campaigns to encourage individuals to engage in treatment as early as possible. Campaigns have emphasized the treatability of depression. There is no need to suffer: come forward and get help.

These are important messages as we certainly need mental health conditions to be de-stigmatized to ensure that everyone who is experiencing these problems feels comfortable coming forward in the way they would with any physical health condition. However, these campaigns tend to present a rather simplistic message. They present depression as a relatively singular entity and treatment as straightforward and typically effective. Depression is a "treatable condition" implies that it usually, if not always, gets better with treatment. Promoting this is certainly understandable. If you want people who might otherwise be reluctant to present for treatment to come forward, you want to provide hope: things are simple and the outcome will be good.

However, is this realistically the case? You don't need to dig very far into any of the literature surrounding depression to soon get the impression that this promotion may not necessarily be so. Depression is certainly extremely common. Whether it is a straightforward condition, or even whether it is really one condition at all, is far less clear.

What is even less clear is how straightforward and effective the treatment will be. There are a variety of effective treatments for depression which will be explored in the following chapters. However, how these treatments are selected for an individual patient and whether they are likely to work or not are certainly much more complex issues. Many patients presenting with depression will have an excellent response, get well, and get back on with their lives. Ideally, this would be the case for everybody. However, it is not. It is well-established that a significant proportion of patients with depression will struggle to get better with standard treatments and some will go many years trying to find the pathway to recovery.

Why is this the case? For some, it will be because their depression is complicated. They might have other physical or mental health problems that impede their progress. In others, there will be psychological or life factors that continue to weigh them down. They might continue to work in a stressful or traumatic environment, they might be stuck in a dysfunctional relationship or carry emotional scars from their childhood or previous life events. However, in some patients, it might just be that the treatments they receive are not good enough.

The medications which are used to treat depression can be wonderful for some patients but in others are useless or cause troublesome side effects. Modern treatment of depression rarely goes far beyond medication. If it does, it might include some limited forms of psychological treatment and occasionally electroconvulsive therapy (modern shock therapy) for the most severely unwell. However, as you will see in the following chapters, good treatment of depression can, and should, include more than this. Treatment should be holistic: address patients' lifestyle, their exercise, their patterns of thought, and their relationships. It should consider a range of potential physical treatments that go beyond standard antidepressant medication. For example, transcranial magnetic stimulation (TMS) has been comprehensively proven to be effective, but its uptake remains patchy, held back in places by the traditional biases of clinicians wedded to doing psychotherapy or prescribing drugs.

Fortunately, the future for patients with depression seems much brighter. There are a range of novel treatments that are being actively developed to help in the management of depression. Some of these are already part of clinical treatment. TMS and forms of the drug ketamine are increasingly becoming more routinely used. Novel drugs, novel forms of psychological treatment and a range of device-based therapies, stimulating the brain from within and from without, are being explored, developed, and in some cases increasingly used. Hopefully reading the following chapters will not just give you an understanding of where we are with the treatment of depression now, but how these emerging treatments are changing things and will continue to do so over the following years.

I would like to make a little bit of a disclaimer. This book is not a textbook, nor is it a guide to learn how to diagnose or treat depression. In reading the pages to follow, you may well recognize many elements of your life or history. I am sure much will also be different and even potentially jarring to your experiences. If you are struggling with depression, hopefully you will learn some things that you can use to help guide your journey going forward.

What I would like most of all, however, is that you can get out of this book, a sense of hope. That you can come to an understanding that the treatment of depression is changing, and changing in a good way. That the treatments that are being developed will increase the options open to you. That as these options expand, your chance of recovery will grow. That you can access effective treatments without significant side-effects, which will support you in your path to recovery. I would also hope that you come away from this with a sense that there are smart and innovative people out there working on these solutions. That what we have now will in no way reflect what the options look like in five, ten or twenty years' time.

The book is divided into several sections. The first chapter begins with an introduction to depression, what it really is, what people experiencing depression describe, how it is diagnosed and what we understand to be its causes. This is followed by several chapters describing how depression is commonly treated right now. There is a chapter on the standard use of antidepressant medications and a second chapter exploring the drug treatments that are tried when standard medications don't work: an all-too-common problem. There are also chapters on talking treatments or psychotherapy and electroconvulsive therapy.

From this point, the book becomes more future focused. This look into the future begins with an in-depth look at the use of transcranial magnetic stimulation, a treatment being used increasingly now and that very much looks like it will have considerable impact in the years to come. I also spend time reviewing a series of other forms of brain stimulation which vary from being very close to clinical use to being quite experimental. I then turn to some novel forms of drug treatment. We will spend a chapter exploring the use of ketamine, an anesthetic agent commonly referred to as a horse tranquilizer, and a chapter exploring the rapidly emerging field of psychedelic assisted psychotherapy.

Through this book, I hope you will come to gain a deeper understanding of what depression is, how it is treated now, and how it is likely to be treated in the years to come. I hope this is a valuable journey.

# 1

# WHAT IS DEPRESSION?

**"I** REALLY JUST DON'T want to be alive. It's not like I would do it, that would be too terrible for my parents. I just don't want to go on living. Every time I go to bed I hope I don't wake up." So began the first conversation I had with Steven. At the time he was 25. Single, living in a share house and trying to hold onto a mundane part time job. He had dropped out of his engineering degree the year before, after spending too many years postponing exams, withdrawing from subjects, hoping to somehow find a way to get through. This was not to be, the black dog was too pervasive and too persistent. For years he had felt like this: unmotivated, miserable, exhausted, as if he had run a marathon following just a trip to the local shops. He struggled to sleep at night but spent days at a time in bed. He had lost interest in food, in hobbies and in friends, and worst of all was that omnipresent sense of hopelessness. It seemed like this was all there was to be, for now and forever. No wonder life did not seem worth living.

This is depression. Steven first felt its dangerous grip as a teenager at age 16. He was doing well at school, had a close relationship with his parents and younger sister and had a number of decent school friends. Life was not bad at all until it was. He struggled for a couple of months, but not like he was struggling now. He kept going to school and although his grades suffered, he put on a brave face, unsure what was going on. Then, relatively suddenly, just as it had appeared from nowhere, back away it seemed to go. Day by day, everything slowly got easier.

A few years later, the depression returned, and this time was different. This time it did not go away by itself. In fact, it stayed and just got worse over time. Steven saw a university counsellor for a few months until the end of the year but then did not go back. He wasn't really sure why but felt like it had just not helped. So, he struggled on by himself. He was embarrassed by his academic decline but did not want anyone to know how he was feeling, what was dragging him down. These problems just did not feel like something you talked to someone about, not in his social circle. At this point, things had got way beyond talking to someone. He could see how far his life had come off the rails and was both shocked and dismayed by this. His family clearly were too and had pushed and pushed him to get some help—so he eventually did. He wanted help, but what he also desperately wanted, understandably so, was some understanding. He needed to know what had gone wrong with him, what was going on, what had he done wrong? And perhaps most critically, was there anything he could do to get his old life back?

So, what was going on? Given that you are reading a book on depression, it is probably a decent guess to assume this is the answer to what was afflicting Steven. If you drew this conclusion, you are right. However, although it is easy to call it depression, it is much harder to really understand what this means because depression is a problem of the most perplexing and complex of organs, the human brain. In keeping with the remarks of the introduction, we are considering depression to be a clinical entity, a significant and typically disabling condition, and not as a troublesome period of sadness which comes and goes. Steven's situation certainly seems to meet this standard.

So, if we are considering depression as a clinical entity, what does that entail? Mental health professionals diagnose patients presenting with depression as having a Major Depressive Episode or a Major Depressive Disorder. A major depressive episode is defined as episode of depression which has extended in time for more than two weeks and is characterized by the patient experiencing a variety of specific typical depressive symptoms. Essentially, depression is a disorder of mood: patients experience a profound change in the pervasive nature of their emotional experience. Commonly, patients just feel persistently sad. They lack the variation and rhythms of normal emotional experience and feel unhappy and frequently tearful. This is not the only element of the emotional experience of patients with depression, however. Many patients with depression, especially when it is severe, describe no longer really feeling sad but rather experiencing a profound absence of emotional experience. They just feel nothing. For many, this is even more disturbing than feeling persistently sad. A capacity to experience emotion directly connects us to the world around us. It provides motivation for action—we do things to seek pleasure, to avoid pain or worry or hurt. Emotion provides the necessary fuel for social interaction while profound absence of emotional experience leads those suffering from depression to increasingly socially disengage.

The second profound emotional symptom of depression is referred to as *anhedonia*. Anhedonia is a term that originates from the Greek words 'an' which means without and 'hēdonē,' which means pleasure. Patients experiencing anhedonia lack the capacity to have pleasurable emotional experiences. These might be in the context of social relationships, hobbies, exercise or any other life experiences that individuals usually engage in that lead to positive feelings. Clearly if someone cannot experience positive emotional responses to the things that they usually enjoy they will be more likely to stop doing anything that provides them with positive rewards. This is part of the vicious negative cycle of depression: as someone becomes increasingly depressed, the nature of their symptoms produces behavioral and social changes that are likely to further exacerbate their depression. They are not enjoying things, so they stop doing them. They stop seeing people, they stop exercising, and they increasingly withdraw. This exacerbates a sense of isolation, of worthlessness, and loneliness.

These negative thoughts and others of guilt, hopelessness, or helplessness are also characteristic symptoms of clinical depression. Depression changes the way people think about themselves, the world around them and their future. Previously optimistic individuals suddenly find themselves seeing everything in the completely opposite way. They blame themselves for things that go wrong but accept no credit for anything that goes right. They feel that they are at fault, for their illness and really for any other bad thing that happens. Perhaps with most impact, they often just cannot see a way out of their current situation. This hopelessness often leads to thoughts that they might be better off dead and in some cases to actual thoughts and plans for suicide. There is often a direct connection between thoughts of hopelessness, that something cannot be done, or there is no way forward, and the idea that the only solution is to end one's life.

As distressing and disabling as the symptoms are, they are only part of the picture that patients with depression face. As well as the emotional symptoms of depression, patients can experience a variety of other cognitive and physical manifestations. A frequently distressing symptom is impaired sleep. Some patients with depression lie awake for hours trying to fall asleep whereas others wake repeatedly during the night and others wake early in the morning at three, four or five a.m., profoundly awake and not able to get back to sleep. Regardless of the time of night, insomnia provides hours of time to think, to worry and ruminate, never a good thing when you are already distressed, sad, and possibly anxious. It is worth noting that some patients have the opposite experience. They sleep a great deal more than they normally would but wake without any sense of relief or satisfaction. Often, when they wake up they feel the same degree of tiredness as they did before they went to bed.

This is similar to the experience of crying. Most people who are not depressed, when they cry, feel some sense of relief. They can feel calmer or soothed. People with depression do not experience this. Tears do not lead to relief or anything good at all. The sense of sadness and despair just hangs there, unchanged.

Anxiety is a very common co-occurrence faced by people with depression. This might be situational: for example, patients are just highly anxious about going out of the house or interacting socially, but it can also be generalized: patients can worry about everything, constantly, all day long. Anxiety involves worrying thoughts, but it also involves the emotional experience and usually distressing physical symptoms. Anxious patients often feel their heart racing, they feel sweaty, lightheaded, dizzy, or short of breath. They can experience tingling and numbness in their arms and legs as well as the typical butterflies in the stomach which can develop into profound nausea. In its most intense and acute form, anxiety can present as a panic attack. During a panic attack, anxiety escalates rapidly, usually over minutes. The patient's physical symptoms are so intense that they might think they are going to die. Patients having a panic attack for the first time often present to an emergency department, convinced that they are having a heart attack.

The experience of anxiety can vary quite a lot across a patient's journey through depression. Some patients become quite anxious when relatively mildly depressed. As their depression worsens, the anxiety might grow. However, the opposite can happen: for some patients, when depression is at its worst, the anxiety fades. They get into a state of being so depressed that they just do not care anymore. They do not have to worry about dying because that would be a relief, not a problem.

Whether they are anxious or not, patients with depression often have significant changes in their desire to eat food. Depression commonly causes a profound lack of interest in food, a loss of appetite, and loss of any sense of pleasure associated with food. Patients with depression can lose large amounts of weight, often very quickly. However, they can also experience the opposite. Sometimes patients have an increased appetite or strong urges to binge eat or consume unhealthy "comfort" foods. Eating this way often exacerbates a sense of guilt or impacts on one's self-esteem.

### Common Symptoms of Depression

- Depressed mood, persistent sadness, tearfulness
- Markedly diminished interest in activities
- Loss of pleasure from almost all activities
- Significant weight loss (not when dieting) or gain
- Decrease or increase in appetite
- Slowed thoughts and a reduction of physical movement
- Problems with sleeping enough or sleeping too much
- Fatigue/loss of energy
- Feelings of worthlessness or excessive/inappropriate guilt
- Diminished ability to think/concentrate or indecisiveness, a cloudiness of thought
- Loss of libido
- Increased anxiety
- Agitation or restlessness
- A sense of dread
- Recurrent thoughts of death, recurrent suicidal ideation or suicide attempt or plan

Another frequently disabling symptom of depression is its impact on concentration, thinking and memory. Patients will frequently find that they struggle to hold information in mind for even relatively short periods of time. When reading they find by the end of a paragraph, that they are struggling to recall the context for what they have just read and need to return to go over the same material multiple times. They might find that more complex plots in television programs or movies are just too hard to follow. This can profoundly affect work or occupational performance and often exacerbates the motivational problems they already experience. The world of their experiences progressively contracts: they engage less and less in previously meaningful day-to-day activities.

The last symptom I want to highlight is that of lethargy. Regardless of whether they sleep too much or sleep too little, patients with depression almost always experience a profound lack of energy. For some, this is experienced as tiredness: they just feel a constant need to sleep no matter how much they have done so, but for others it is a different feeling. They just lack the energy to do things. It is like there is no petrol in the tank and the car just will not go.

Given the range of these symptoms that patients can experience, it is no wonder that patients with depression can be profoundly disabled by their condition. Many patients with depression struggle in extraordinarily brave ways to maintain roles: to go to work, to study or to care for their families. Some patients can maintain functioning in one area of their life but not others. They might be able to maintain functioning at work, but they come home, eat and fall straight into bed, remaining there for 12 hours until they have to get up and return to work, or for the entire weekend. Steven managed to function for short periods of time in a relatively undemanding part time job, but just could not do more—study or more prolonged periods of work were just too overwhelming. For some patients, even his amount of functioning is not possible: the depression is just too severe. They are unable to maintain any meaningful degree of activity and can be bedridden. At its most severe, patients with depression can get to a point of completely losing the capacity to function. Some patients will find even the basic acts of eating and drinking overwhelming, and it is a struggle just to survive.

When Steven presented for assessment, it was important, not just to explore the symptoms of depression itself, but to explore whether there were symptoms of related conditions, other than depression itself, things that could better explain his presentation. There are a number of conditions that can look like depression, producing similar or overlapping symptoms (see the table on the next page). Perhaps the most important clinically is bipolar disorder, what used to be called manic depression.

Bipolar disorder is a condition, much less common than depression itself, where patients experience episodes of depression, often many over a lifetime. They, however, also experience periods of profound mood elevation: called mania or hypomania depending on how severe they are. These superficially sound pleasant and productive. Patients can be euphoric, energized, do not need to sleep, and have lots of ideas. However, it can also be very unpleasant, dysfunctional, and destructive. Euphoria often morphs to profound irritability; the increased energy is wasted as the patient bounces from uncompleted task to uncompleted task and the ideas can become delusions: false beliefs that the patient has profound powers or is special in some very important way. Patients during mania can be very impulsive, making decisions and acting in ways very much out of character. This can have profound personal, financial, and occupational consequences with the patient left to pick up the pieces of a damaged life as they recover from an episode. Recovery is also complicated by the fact that a manic episode usually ends with a depressive one: often a devastating and then long persistent come down.

If someone presents with depression for the first time, who has never had any evidence of mania or hypomania, it is impossible to know whether they have depression or bipolar disorder. However, the former is much more common, and this will be how the patient will be treated. If there is any evidence of periods of mood elevation in the past, this needs to be explored as the treatment of these conditions does differ. Most importantly, the common antidepressant medications used for depression can cause a variety of problems in patients with bipolar disorder and are best avoided.

| OTHER CONDITIONS FOR CONSIDERATION IN A PATIENT WITH DEPRESSION ||
| Condition | Comments |
| --- | --- |
| **Bipolar disorder** | Distinct periods of mood elevation as well as depression |
| **Cyclothymic disorder** | Prolonged periods of mild depression or mania (hypomania) |
| **Mood disorder due to a medical condition** | Depression directly brought on by a medical condition such as hypothyroidism |
| **Premenstrual dysphoric disorder** | Severe dysphoria, irritability, or mood swings for a week prior to the onset of menses and finishing a few days after the onset of menses |
| **Persistent depressive disorder (dysthymia)** | This describes a state of prolonged (2 years plus) depression of somewhat less severity than would be seen in true depression |
| **Substance / medication induced mood disorder** | Depression brought about by the use of illicit or prescription drugs |

The clinical form of depression that we are talking about is actually an extraordinarily common condition. The reality of this, and its impact on society, is finally being recognized although the resources dedicated to understanding depression and treating patients who suffer from it still lags shamefully behind the resources dedicated to much less common physical health conditions. Studies have repeatedly identified that between 5% to 10% of the population experience depression during any one year and about 15% of the population will experience an episode at some time during their life. Depression does not discriminate. It is a condition that affects people across the full socio-economic spectrum, across cultural groups and ages. Depression frequently presents for the first time when people are quite young but is also a common occurrence in the elderly.

Why does depression occur? Steven wanted to know this—why does it happen, and especially why did it happen to him? This is the question for which there is definitively not a straightforward answer. Modern psychiatry tends to regard depression as a "multifactorial" illness. This means that across the vast number of people who develop depression, and typically within an individual person as well, there will be multiple things that potentially contribute to the development of the condition. These factors range widely across the domains of biology, psychology, social—cultural and even environmental influences.

From a biological or physical perspective, there is clearly some degree of genetic contribution to the likelihood that an individual will develop a depressive illness. If your parents have depression, or multiple other family members, you will be more likely to develop the illness yourself than someone who does not have this family background. However, you are only *more likely* to develop depression, it is by no means genetically inevitable. It would be a reasonable question to ask how we can be sure about this. People who share genes also tend to share a lot of other things in life: they are likely to come from the same socioeconomic conditions, siblings will have shared experiences of parenting and so on. It may be that depression runs in families for other, non-genetic, reasons. This may be the case, and probably is for many. However, studies which have explored the likelihood of depression developing in twins (who will share all or only some of the same genes depending on whether they are identical) strongly suggest a role for genes. This is also suggested by another line of research: the study of depression in individuals raised away from their natural parents due to adoption. A very large Swedish study published in 2018 found that individuals raised by adoptive parents had an increased risk of depression if this was seen in their biological family.*

Beyond genetics, a considerable body of research has explored the actual brain factors that might underpin the development of depression. For many decades, this research focused on the possibility that depression relates to abnormalities in the levels or function of certain neurochemicals in the brain, and especially the neurotransmitters serotonin and noradrenaline. What are these? To understand this requires a little understanding of how the brain works. The brain contains a fairly astonishing number of nerve cells (also called neurons): on average about 80-100 billion. These nerve cells have a variety of connections, miniature biological 'wires' that they use to connect to one another. These wires make an even more astonishing, in fact, inconceivable high number of connections with one another, possibly more than 100 trillion in total. The wires from one cell do not join up with the wires of the next one, but they come very, very close. There are small gaps between these wires, called synapses. One of the cells will pass a message to the next cell across this synapse by releasing a chemical messenger—we call this a neurotransmitter. The neurotransmitter passes across the synapse and attaches itself to a receptor on the next nerve cell, fastening itself like a key might in a lock. This triggers chemical and electrical activity in the second nerve cell, passing along the signal.

There are lots of different neurotransmitters in the brain, each with a different type of lock to bind to and each with a different role. Serotonin and noradrenaline are not the most common neurotransmitters in the brain, far from it, but they do seem to punch above their weight in terms of importance of action. They are found at the end of a relatively small number of nerve cells, but these cells have unusual properties. The cells tend to be found deep down in the brain, in a small number of concentrated areas. Their wires, however, pass widely around the brain (and down the spinal cord). They pass into most of the areas of the brain that are involved in complex thinking as well as generation and regulation of emotion. In these areas, they can tune up or tune down activity in other nerve cells. In this way, a small number of nerve cells have the ability to regulate or influence activity in widespread areas or circuits within the brain.

Given this, it would make sense to think that changes in serotonin and/or noradrenaline could cause depression. Change these and you could alter many functions of the brain, and as we have discussed, depression certainly involves the disruption of lots of different brain functions. This was not the reason why serotonin and noradrenaline were implicated in depression, however. The reason for this was a little more straightforward.

As we will discuss in the next chapter, the first drugs that could be used to treat depression were discovered in the late 1950s and early 1960s. Although these drugs were not developed purposefully to change serotonin and noradrenaline to relieve depression, it was soon realized that their actions were to increase these neurotransmitters in the brain. This led to a somewhat inevitable, but not necessarily correct assumption, that if increasing these neurotransmitters helps depression, then the disorder must be caused by a lack of serotonin or noradrenaline to begin with. This seductive idea really misled psychiatry and neuroscience research for many decades and lead to a considerable mythology around depression and its causes: especially the so called "serotonin hypothesis" of depression.

Let's make this clear: depression is not caused by not having enough serotonin in the brain. This was a seductively simple explanation for depression and one that was ideally suited to help to promote the sales of antidepressants, but is just not true. Research has clearly failed to find a consistent deficit of serotonin in the brains of patients with depression. Serotonin is involved in the condition in some way, but the reality of the disorder is much more complicated than this simplistic idea. This idea has been used as an effective sales pitch for the pharmaceutical industry and mislead the decent part of a generation of depression research.

On a more positive note, even if untrue, the idea that depression was caused by a chemical deficiency was able to be used to help reduce a lot of the stigma associated with depression. Just as diabetes was caused by not enough insulin (which could be corrected), so might depression have a chemical explanation (also corrected with the new "wonder drugs"). This was clearly misleading but perhaps not more so, and in a less damaging way, than some of the social ideas about depression that blamed the character of individuals for what they were experiencing.

So, what do we know now about what is going on in the brain of a patient with depression? One way to think about the biology of depression is that it is a condition where there is a disruption in the complex interaction between areas of the brain or the networks that bind these together. Modern neuroimaging (brain scanning) studies have clearly identified changes in activity levels in multiple brain areas in patients with depression. There are areas of the brain which consistently fail to show the same levels of blood flow or metabolic activity (the consumption of the energy required for normal brain function) as they do in individuals without depression. However, there is also a corresponding but very different set of brain areas where blood flow or energy consumption is substantially increased. These changes have been seen in many brain imaging studies and they mostly return to normal when patients recover from the illness, regardless of the treatment used to produce this improvement.

In parallel with this research, neuroimaging and other modern neuroscience studies have been used to help discover that there are quite defined networks in the brain. These networks involve a number of brain regions that work together to help the brain perform certain tasks or are simultaneously active when somebody is in a particular state of thought. There is a clear overlap between the areas of the brain that have been shown to be abnormally active in patients with depression and some of these well-defined networks. For example, patients with depression typically show a lack of activation of networks involved in concentration and other aspects of deliberate cognitive effort. This is clearly consistent with the experience of patients who struggle to focus and with other aspects of thinking. Studies have also shown a significant increase in activation in brain networks associated with self-focused thought; this is believed to underpin the persistent negative ruminative thoughts that patients with depression typically experience.

## Functional Brain Imaging: Sorting the Myth From Reality

Modern forms of brain imaging, especially functional magnetic resonance imaging (fMRI) have taken on an almost mystical aura in regards to their capacity to unlock the secrets of the brain. A seemingly endless series of studies are publicized in the general media, presumably at the behest of enthusiastic university public relations departments, informing us how the latest study has demonstrated the critical role of brain region 'X' in a certain brain function. All understanding seemingly just awaits the creativity of researchers.

The truth is a little less impressive. Imaging studies do tend to indicate which areas might be involved in which types of thinking—these areas "light up" when someone is scanned doing a task of interest. However, they do not provide any concrete evidence that any one area is necessary for the task in question. Amongst the series of brain 'blobs' that light up on scanning, some may well be essential but others are likely to be epiphenomena, just secondary effects. It is usually not possible to tell which are which.

There is another major limitation of these methods worth mentioning. Generally speaking, these forms of scanning scan can show interesting differences when comparing multiple scans from different people: for example, differences between the "averaged" brains of 20 people with depression compared to 20 people without. However, this does not mean we can look at the scan of a single depressed patient and really say anything at all from this observation. The scans themselves are just too 'noisy' and inaccurate to allow this. This is despite what some will have you believe. Every now and then I hear about a clinician who is scanning patients' brains and using the scans to say something about their diagnosis and treatment; the best I can say about this is that it is a high tech version of phrenology, the 18th century practice of inferring mental characteristics by reading bumps on the skull. The scans and interpretations are often very impressive indeed and add a veneer of science to something that usually seems very unscientific. However, the technology is just not up to this yet and money should be much more appropriately and productively spent elsewhere. If your doctor proposes to take a pretty multi-colored picture of your brain to diagnose your depression, it is time to consider finding another doctor.

What underpins the disruption of these brain areas and networks? This is a much more difficult question to answer and one for which we do not currently have a satisfactory answer. It is possible, and I would think is likely, that there is not a single process that does this but potentially quite a number. It is possible that a disruption in a variety of neurochemicals or hormones in the brain could disrupt the delicate balance of activity levels between brain regions resulting in differing individuals developing a similar disruption of broader brain network activity.

In other words, the disruption of these brain networks would be "a final common pathway" through which multiple mechanisms could ultimately produce a similar clinical pattern. For example, some patients with depression might have a disruption of functioning in their serotonin system (not likely a simple reduction in serotonin). In other patients, the primary biological mechanism might involve a change in function of the noradrenaline neurotransmitter or perhaps dopamine, another chemical involved in widespread regulatory activity in the brain. In other patients, it might involve a change in gamma-aminobutyric acid (GABA). GABA is actually one of the most ubiquitous neurotransmitters in the brain, found in about 30% of the connections between nerve cells, and studies have suggested that GABA levels are reduced in patients with depression and increased with successful antidepressant treatment.

In other patients, the primary disruption may not be in these typical neurotransmitters but could be in some of the other chemicals in the brain. For example, the neuro-steroid hormones that help regulate activity of GABA and other neurotransmitters. In others, the fault might not be neurochemical at all. For example, a mild traumatic head injury might disrupt some of the critical connections between brain areas disrupting the network balance. In others, sustained hardship or traumatic life events might result in changes mediated through the stress response or even inflammation.

This reminds us that depression is clearly not a purely biological illness. It is something that results from a complex interplay between an individual's psychological makeup, life experiences and biological wiring. There are many ways that life experiences, from before we are born, to those during childhood and then during our adult life, can affect the brain and how it functions. Many patients who experience depression have experienced profoundly traumatic events in their early lives or adulthood. Our personality and coping styles, themselves shaped by all of our biology, parenting, and life experiences, will determine how we evaluate the events of our lives and the impact that these have on us.

This complex interaction ultimately determines who we are but also the likelihood of whether we will suffer from mental health conditions, such as depression. Psychiatry has struggled with these concepts for many years. Throughout much of the previous century, depression was divided into two broad categories, often referred to as *endogenous* or *reactive* depression. Endogenous depression was a disorder of biology: it proposed that you would develop depression because of an inherent biological process. Reactive depression, in contrast, would develop, as the name implies, as a reaction to some trauma or other life event. Fortunately, we have now moved beyond this simplistic split.

The type of research study that helped convince me that this was a blatantly inadequate way of thinking about depression involved researchers exploring the relationship between adverse life events—traumas—and the likelihood that individuals would develop depression. In this type of study, researchers use questionnaires that aim to quantify how many difficult life events patients had experienced in a defined period of time preceding an episode of depression. The researchers were interested in exploring whether negative life events—like the loss of a loved one or divorce—were more common in the time prior to a depressive episode compared to other periods in a patient's life or to the experience of similar people who had not developed depression. They then asked the question as to whether patients experiencing an episode of depression reported more negative life events prior to the episode than individuals in the same communities and of the same age.

This was certainly the case: overall, negative life events are clearly more common in the time prior to the development of depression. However, the results were somewhat more complicated than that. Negative life events were clearly much more common before an episode of depression that was the first episode of depression experienced by an individual during their life. Negative life events seem to be an important trigger for the first time someone would develop depression. However, although patients would commonly report negative life events during subsequent relapses of depression later in life, they did not report these more commonly than healthy, age-matched individuals. Negative life events did not seem to be relevant in increasing the likelihood of, or triggering of, these recurrences of depression.

This leaves us with a much more complex model. Challenging life events appeared to be of significant importance in the onset of depression, in potentially triggering the first episode. However, after the first, or perhaps a second episode, the illness seems to take on a life of its own with recurrences not necessarily being nearly as directly connected to external influences. If we use the old language, this would imply that most patients initially have an episode of reactive depression but then subsequent episodes are endogenous, a conceptualization that doesn't really make a lot of sense.

What makes more sense is to imagine patients as having some degree of vulnerability, presumably related to their genetics, early life experiences, or trauma. The first episode of depression is then triggered by one or multiple stressful life experiences. Actually experiencing an episode of depression produces some degree of change in the nature of the individual's brain. Even when they fully recover, this experience of having had depression lays down a predisposition or vulnerability for future episodes, which can occur either triggered by future life events or out of the blue.

There are numerous psychological theories of depression occupying reams of library and bookshelf space. It is not within the scope of this book to review all or even a representative proportion of these. In simplistic terms, many people with depression have some form of vulnerability in the way in which they interact with the world or appraise the circumstances of their daily lives. For example, some people who are likely to develop depression tend to judge themselves harshly and have an "external locus of control". This means they attribute anything good that happens to them as occurring by chance or resulting from events outside of their control, and anything bad as being a result of their own personal characteristics. Other people have fixed patterns of thought such that they "automatically" bring negative thoughts to mind, often repeatedly and consistently over time. Suffice to say, the management of depression, as will be discussed in the following chapters, can only sensibly progress if these issues are understood and a comprehensive management plan developed to help address them. There will be patients where the presence and recurrence of depression seems driven by, and interdependent with, these psychological factors. There will be other patients where the experience of recurrent depression itself, affects their outlook and the way they see the world, the relationship switched around the other way. Regardless of these factors, depression does seem to become embedded in the brain in some intransient and meaningful way. Its tendency to recur, increasingly independently of life events, emphasizes the degree to which there seems to be a form of biological imprinting, regardless of the underlying triggers or causes.

Adopting this model, of depression as a disorder of disrupted activity in specific networks around the brain triggered by variable underlying causes, has a number of really important implications for the way we think about how existing treatments work and about how we might develop new ways of helping patients. For one, it explains why existing treatments are not always successful. As will be explored in Chapter 3, commonly used antidepressant medications frequently do not relieve depression. Modern antidepressants are fairly specifically targeted to one or more neurotransmitter systems. If an individual patient's depression has been triggered by changes in noradrenaline, it would make sense they do not respond to an antidepressant that affects serotonin and vice versa. It is also possible that the medication may make changes to the functioning in the neurotransmitter system, but this may not automatically fix the disruption of network activity that results from the original trigger or cause.

Perhaps more importantly, this network model suggests a variety of new ways that might be used to modify brain activity with therapeutic intent. As will be discussed at some length in this book, a profoundly alternative approach is to try directly targeting activity in the brain regions that were shown to be disrupted in depression with various alternative forms of stimulation. These may be forms of electrical or magnetic stimulation applied to particular brain regions in the relevant networks to try to restore more normal network functioning. This could also involve the use of specific cognitive training—involving patients in targeted puzzles and brain training activities—to try to activate critical brain regions without external stimulation. Activation of specific networks in this way requires a sophisticated understanding of the brain regions involved in depression and how they interact. Presumably, the best form of stimulation is going to be targeted at critical hubs in this network where inducing local changes can have flown effects around the network.

There is an alternative approach to understanding network-based brain activity that is not as focused on brain structures, but instead, is based on trying to decode the language of the brain. The "language" that allows regions of the brain to communicate with one another, often at distance, is the pattern of rhythmic firing of nerve cells. Nerve cells do not fire by themselves. Instead, in local areas of the brain, groups of nerve cells typically fire together and fire repeatedly in the same rhythm. Distributed areas of the brain that work together in a particular network coordinate also their action by having nerve cells across these different regions fire at the same time and at the same rhythm.

The pattern of these "brainwaves" can be detected and recorded using electroencephalography (EEG) equipment: EEG records electrical activity on the surface of the scalp arising from the firing of brain cells in the underlying brain. EEG recordings show that the rhythms that underpin brain activity in patients with depression tend to differ from those in healthy individuals. These recordings also show that the frequencies that individuals use for this long-range communication tend to differ. They will typically be in the same range, for example, in the theta range between four and 8 Hz, but each individual's frequency of preference will be slightly different. Mine might be 5.1 Hz and yours might be 5.7 Hz. Understanding how brain rhythms differ in patients compared to healthy individuals allows us to potentially apply forms of stimulation that are not necessarily highly targeted but allow us to manipulate the frequency of communication between multiple brain regions and to try to restore this to a more normal pattern. This will be explored further in Chapter 8.

So does all this theory help us to understand Steven better? Or to provide him an explanation for his troubles? We do have an increasingly sophisticated understanding of depression, but our capacity to apply this to tease apart what is going on for individual patients remains frustratingly limited. We can provide patients with a model that is probably more accurate than "you don't have enough serotonin," but we still need to talk in generalities and hypotheses. This, unfortunately, is likely to remain the case for some time. The resources spent on trying to understand depression and other mental health conditions are minuscule compared to those spent on unlocking the secrets of physical health conditions, despite the disproportionate impact of depression and the overwhelming complexities of the brain and mind.

In conclusion, the depression that we are addressing in this book is a profound clinical condition that is both extremely common and frequently highly disabling. Depression manifests itself in a variety of ways but typically patients experience a range of symptoms that impact their capacity to experience normal emotions, think clearly, have energy and motivation, sleep and eat normally, and undertake all of their normal daily activities. We don't fully understand what causes depression, but all the available evidence suggests that this is a complex condition that develops through an interaction between the biology of the brain and an extensive range of life experiences and social circumstances. We are, however, increasingly understanding aspects of the neurobiology of depression and this is progressively enhancing our capacity to develop treatments. Before we address these, we'll be spending the next couple of chapters exploring what is currently done to help patients with depression—and why we need to go beyond this current state of play.

# 2

# FROM FREUD TO FACEBOOK: PSYCHOTHERAPY IN THE MANAGEMENT OF DEPRESSION

THIS IS A book predominately about the biological management of depression: of drugs and devices. But no consideration of this topic would be complete without addressing the role that psychological interventions have in the management of depression. There are many tomes covering this area: in this chapter, I do not promise to replace or even summarize these. I do, however, wish to give a practical view as to how psychological interventions can fit into the management of the more severe end of the depressive spectrum: to find some useful middle ground between those who think that therapy and social change should be the cure for all and the view that depression is a biomedical illness with purely physical solutions.

Any consideration of the relative role of psychological and biological treatments in the management of depression has to begin with addressing the question of illness severity. The evidence supporting the use of medication clearly suggests that medication is more likely to be effective in more severe depression. As will be addressed in Chapter 3, there is clearly less difference between the effect of placebo and active medication the milder the illness severity. Psychological treatment is somewhat the opposite: it is more likely to be both practical and effective in patients with more mild or moderately severe forms of the illness.

One factor which is critical in both the psychological and biomedical treatment of depression is the strength and quality of the relationships formed between patients and those professionals engaged in their care. Given the complexity of treatment choices (as is hopefully made amply evident in this book) this relationship needs to be a collaborative one. It is of paramount importance that patients are provided with education and are supported to make critical choices about their care. This is clearly no less relevant, and probably more so, when we are examining the situation for patients where initial treatment options have failed to work. Patients under these circumstances may have accumulated the involvement of multiple health care professionals; family doctors, psychologists, psychiatrists, and others, in their care team and it is important that efforts are made to ensure the care provided is coordinated and consistent.

### Psychiatrist, Psychologist or Therapist: Does It Matter?

Psychological therapies can be provided by therapists with a range of professional backgrounds. Psychiatrists are medical doctors who have undertaken specialty training in the treatment of patients with mental health conditions. They are able to prescribe medication and order investigations such as x-rays and blood tests and may choose to also offer psychological treatments. In fact, psychiatrists vary considerably in whether they are predominately focused on providing biological treatments, such as medication, or who mostly provide one or various forms of psychotherapy. There are individuals at either end of the spectrum who just focus on physical treatments or psychological treatments and many who combine both in their clinical practice. Psychologists do not have a biomedical background but are specifically trained in the provision of psychological treatments and so only offer various forms of therapy. Therapists from either discipline will vary in whether they specialize in one form of psychological treatment, and only provide this, or whether they use different forms of therapy depending on the needs of an individual patient.

The importance of a good patient-therapist fit cannot be underestimated. I pretty much always advise patients seeking a therapist that the process is a little like dating. You do not go out on a first date expecting that this person will automatically be "the one." In fact, invest too much hope in that first date and you will probably find a way to muck it up. Meeting a new therapist can be very anxiety provoking. Patients doing so are vulnerable, doubting themselves and often even second-guessing whether they are doing the right thing. Can they really explain how they feel? Is the person judging them? Do they look foolish? I think it is of real importance when undertaking this challenging process that patients do not feel like they have to always "make it work." In reality, it might take several tries to find the right therapist: the person with whom you connect and feel comfortable disclosing your deepest secrets. Therefore, if you do not feel right with the first person, so be it: be prepared to move on. But first, take a moment to reflect. Analyze whether this was just your discomfort with the process: this is certainly a common reaction to seeing a therapist for the first time. If, however, the issues are with the individual, you just do not feel that this person is the right fit, do not feel like you have to persevere, keep looking.

The same principle applies to the approach being proposed by the therapist. As we will discuss, not all therapy is equal. In fact, there are many different approaches. Some are more evidence-based than others. In other words, some forms of therapy have been systematically evaluated in clinical trials, in much the same way that a medication or other treatment would be tested. Other forms of therapy, fortunately ones being used much less commonly now, seem to rely more on the faith of the practitioners in the theoretical model underpinning what they do. They believe it works so you should too. Do not be afraid to question what is being proposed: what type of therapy is being offered? What training and experience does the therapist have in this approach? Why is this type of therapy for you right now?

Psychological treatment may well have been recommended or tried when a patient first started to experience depression, often before medication is tried. It commonly will have been tried well before a patient presents with a more challenging depression, one that does not seem to be responding to a variety of treatments. As a clinician it is critical, however, to reconsider what the format, type, and quality of this therapy has been. General supportive psychological care or counselling (what is sometimes referred to as supportive psychotherapy), does have a role in the milder forms of depression. Mild depression has a reasonable chance of spontaneously disappearing, especially with good support.

However, supportive counseling is not a well-supported treatment for more severe forms of depression. If you have being seeing a psychologist and the nature of the time you spend in the sessions is a relatively general discussion of day-to-day issues, chances are that this is what has been provided. Patients receiving this kind of treatment often feel better immediately afterward—they have been listened to, perhaps they have unburdened themselves—but the treatment much less commonly has a lasting beneficial effect. Under these circumstances, it is important to consider alternatives: forms of therapy that are specifically *treatments* for depression. But what are these? *

## Counseling and its Value in Depression

Considerable debate continues over the relative value of various forms of therapy for common disorders such as depression. Recent studies have indicated that there is evidence that counseling can have short term benefits, but these do not seem to persist over time in a meaningful way. One study from the University of Manchester recently summarized data from nine studies involving 1384 patients. This found short-term benefits but the failure of these to persist in the long-term and no effects on the social functioning of patients.

There are, in fact, quite specific forms of psychotherapy that should be used in the treatment of depression and these should be provided by therapists who are specifically and appropriately trained for the provision of these. The application of these therapies is usually guided by a specific manual: the trials that have successfully demonstrated the benefits of

* Cochrane Database Syst Rev. 2011 Sep 7;(9):CD001025. DOI: 10.1002/14651858. CD001025.pub3. Counselling for mental health and psychosocial problems in primary care. Bower P1, Knowles S, Coventry PA, Rowland N.

psychological interventions have generally used manuals describing in detail how the therapy should be conducted and implemented procedures to ensure that therapists follow these accurately. It is unclear how effective these treatments are out in general use if therapists start to diverge from the formally described processes.

There are multiple forms of psychotherapy that have been supported in research studies. Generally, the effects of psychological treatment in most studies could be described as "modest": these therapies work but only in a limited subset of patients: a similar problem to that seen with medication. Recent analyses have not shown substantial differences in effectiveness across a number of types of therapy: they are about as good as each other. It is worth noting, however, that cognitive behavioral therapy (CBT) has been supported by a much greater number of studies than the other options we will discuss.

Before we address these specific forms of therapy, it is worthy of note that although there are times when psychotherapy is presented as a form of treatment that is suitable for everyone, this is certainly not the case. Some will argue that psychotherapy is the answer to the evils of medication treatment, and that it is a safe and effective treatment that should be provided to all patients. However, this is way too simplistic. Psychotherapy is certainly not suitable for everyone. Patients may not be willing to engage in this form of treatment, may not be attuned to the type of therapy being presented, or may be too unwell to meaningfully participate in it. Illness severity is a critical factor. More unwell patients with depression can lack the motivation, energy, or even hope that they need to put the effort in to meaningfully engage. Patients overwhelmed with hopelessness may see the process as pointless. Patients whose depression has affected their concentration and thinking may not be able to focus and concentrate in a way that is required.

Psychological mindedness is a concept that some therapists use when they are considering whether a patient is suitable for psychotherapy. It refers to the ability of someone to be able to reflect on their own internal life or psychological processes. It was originally a concept that applied to forms of Freudian psychoanalytic psychotherapy but generally is useful in thinking about suitability for psychotherapy in general. People will significantly vary in how interested they are in reflecting on their own internal life and they will also vary in their capacity to do so. These factors will clearly have a meaningful impact on whether certain patients are suitable for therapy in general and how suitable they are for specific types of therapy.

Proposing psychotherapy as a widespread solution to the problems with medication also implies the availability of an experienced and skillful workforce. In my experience, gained from asking hundreds of patients about what happens during their therapy, there is dramatic variability in the therapy provided to patients with depression. All too frequently, patients describe receiving supportive counseling, rather than a more depression-specific form of therapy. Geographical distribution of therapists, availability in rural areas, and the cost, remain significant barriers to care.

One solution that has been proposed to make consistent structured therapy available widely is the provision of internet-based therapy, such as internet-based CBT. A number of internet-based therapy systems have been subject to structured research suggesting that they can have value in reducing depressive symptoms. However, this research has predominately focused on mild depression. In addition, internet-based therapy is typically associated with high dropout rates. These issues limit its value to the types of patients we are discussing in this book. Nevertheless, it could prove a useful additional intervention if one-on-one therapy is inaccessible.

So, what are the types of therapy that should be actively considered in treating depression? Clearly, the leading light is CBT. CBT has its roots in several developments in the field of psychology in the 1900s. Behaviorism was first described in the 1920s by individuals such as Skinner and Watson. This proposed that behaviors developed through conditioning: through the effect of the environment on us as individuals, and that thoughts and feelings do not play an active role in determining actions. Mental health conditions could be tackled by directly changing behavior. This was a radically different approach from the predominant mode of psychological therapy used from the early 1900s through to the 1970s and 1980s, psychoanalytical therapy (think of Freud and the couch).

Modern CBT arose from a combination of this early 20th century behaviorism with the emerging field of cognitive therapy in the 1950s and 60s. The 1950s saw the development of what was called rational emotive behavior therapy (REBT) by Albert Ellis: REBT was based on the idea that our emotional state is determined by how we view events, not specifically the events themselves. In the following decade, Aaron Beck developed what was initially called cognitive therapy. Beck was a psychiatrist who typically was engaged in the practice of psychoanalytic psychotherapy. He noted the presence in his depressed patients of so called "automatic thoughts." These were negative thoughts, about the person, their world or the future, which would repeatedly arise in mind. Beck first described how these negative thoughts would go on to influence our feelings and then our behavior: these effects could result then in further negative thoughts. He went on to develop an approach to therapy where the focus was on identifying and challenging these thoughts—very much the basis of modern CBT.

Over subsequent decades, especially as long-term psychoanalytic therapy has waned in popularity, CBT and related techniques have come to dominate psychological approaches to mental health concerns, now much more broadly than depression. CBT is a type of "manualized" therapy. It has also been traditionally presented as a time limited therapy provided over a pre-specified number of sessions. These features have allowed for the implementation of structured clinical trials that were far more problematic with previous forms of less structured and open ended therapies. These have catalyzed the uptake of CBT and provided a considerable degree of legitimacy.

The same features, however, have also fueled criticism. The highly structured format on one hand is criticized for lacking flexibility: of lacking capacity to be tailored to the needs of individual patients. Conversely, therapists implementing CBT outside of clinical trials have been criticized for too loosely following the manualized structure. If they are not following the structure carefully, they will not be providing treatment that has been proven to be effective.

CBT has also been criticized for its general philosophical approach. For example, attributing suffering to the way people evaluate their circumstances ignores the importance of the profound impact of trauma experienced in their lives. Or it ignores the importance of the social environment. People are fundamentally responsible for their suffering, regardless of the societal conditions in which they live. These concerns, however, have not really limited the widespread uptake of CBT or of the many variants or other forms of manualized therapy that have evolved over recent decades.

One of the more prominent alternative approaches to CBT places the central focus not on our thoughts or how we appraise our circumstances, but in the relationships that we have with other people. This is referred to as interpersonal therapy (IP). IP has a basic premise: that depression or other mental health issues arise through problems in interpersonal relationships. These are the focus of the therapy, which has also been formalized in manual form and validated in clinical trials. IP has an interesting backstory. It was initially developed in the 1970s as a form of structured therapy to be applied alongside antidepressant medication in a long-term randomized trial in patients with depression.* The therapy was developed to be explicitly time limited and structured.

IP was developed and based within a medical model of depression. The central concept, which was unusual at the time when psychoanalytic thought and increasingly CBT were predominant, saw depression as a medical condition imposed on the patient and something the patient was not to be blame for. The theory behind IP proposed that individuals could become vulnerable to depression when there were disruptions to, or problems with, interpersonal relationships, such as the death of a loved one, disputes with other people, or social isolation. In contrast, meaningful social relationships and support is protective. Relationships would also be disrupted by depression: thus, there was a reason to focus on these as a cause and an effect of the illness. Although it was first

* Markowitz, J. C., & Weissman, M. M. (2012). Interpersonal psychotherapy: past, present and future. *Clinical psychology & psychotherapy, 19*(2), 99–105. doi:10.1002/cpp.1774

developed back in the 1970s, IP took much longer to spread into popular use than the forms of CBT that came before it. However, this does not reflect the quality of the research evidence which has progressively grown over time and clearly supports its use in the treatment of depression as well as now in other disorders.

Any superficial consideration of the ideas behind CBT and IP will suggest that these are not automatically competing options but therapies that could be offered side by side to different patients or even to the same patient at different times in their lives. A good formulation of a patients' problems may suggest the need to specifically focus on relationships or more on the internal factors which are the main focus of CBT, determining the most appropriate approach to take at any one point in time. It is important to note that these are both quite active forms of therapy. Successful participation will require the patient to actively engage in the therapy process and be willing to examine the role that their thoughts and actions play in underpinning their experience of depression.

Beyond CBT and IP, there are a number of other forms of therapy whose use is also supported by clinical trial evidence. Behavioral activation, a more specifically behavioral approach, problem solving therapy and a brief form of the more traditional psychodynamic psychotherapy all have some support. There is also support for several newer therapy forms of therapy including Acceptance and Commitment therapy (ACT).

### What is a Formulation?

Developing a formulation, alongside making a diagnosis, is considered a cornerstone of psychiatry. A formulation is an attempt to come to an understanding of the factors contributing to the present state of a patient, something that is seen to be complementary to making a formal diagnosis. Whereas a diagnosis asks the clinician to consider how this patient is like others (how do their symptoms fit into a pattern), formulation does the opposite: it is concerned with how the patient is unique. In other words, what are the factors in the patient's past and present that have led them to where they are now? These may be biological/physical, psychological, or social.

By understanding the factors that have contributed to the development of the patient's current condition, an understanding is formed of how the patient is different from other patients who have the same diagnosis. How they, amongst all the patients with depression, for example, are unique. This should then also determine treatment. Understanding the unique elements of a patient's condition allows a treatment plan to be formed, taking into account all the relevant biological, psychological and social factors that have led the person in question to be presenting for treatment at this point in time.

I have mentioned psychodynamic or psychoanalytic psychotherapy several times. This is the modern day treatment that has evolved from Freudian psychoanalysis. Psychodynamic therapy remains an approach with a long-term time horizon: the expectation is not of rapid change. Patients engage in unstructured therapy sessions which are very much the opposite of the manual driven therapies we have discussed so far. Patients undertaking this form of therapy speak about anything that comes to mind and the therapist's role, in part, is to understand and interpret the significance of what arises in therapy to help the patient come to a deeper understanding of their psychological processes. It is expected that the patient will develop an attachment to the therapist that will allow them to work through various significant relationships from their past. Dysfunctional relationships from the past get played out in the safe space of the therapeutic relationship, allowing the patient to develop both deeper emotional and intellectual insight. There are many variations on psychodynamic therapy that have evolved over time, but these all have lessened in prominence as the approach in general has fallen from favor over time.

The decline of analytic therapy has in part related to questions over its effectiveness and whether this can ever be established in meaningful trials. It is certainly hard to imagine patients willingly participating in a randomized trial of therapy conducted multiple times per week and potentially for several years (as this type of therapy is) if the trial involved a chance of receiving some form of placebo treatment, whatever this might be. Additionally, the cost, and complexity of the treatment itself, the increasing availability of alternative therapeutic options, and the growing emphasis on biological treatments in psychiatry have all played a role in its decline. A rear-guard action has formed around the use of more time limited forms of dynamic therapy. Treatment is provided using the same principles but within a limited number of sessions and by necessity with a more proactive or focused approach. There is increasingly clinical trial evidence for this approach in the treatment of depression. Whether used in a time limited or the more traditional way, dynamic therapy probably is most useful when depression is underpinned by clearly problematic relationships or events in the past and the patient has a quite specific interest in wanting to explore and understand the impact of these. In addition, it can be a lifesaving and profoundly important intervention for individuals struggling with depression who have experienced substantial early life trauma and where treatment by necessity requires a long-term approach focused on how this trauma has impacted the development of an individual's view of themselves, as well as the way they engage in relationships.

Mindfulness-based cognitive therapy (MBCT) is another form of therapy worthy of specific attention, particularly given the popularity of various forms of mindfulness in the community in general. This is a relatively recently developed approach, first proposed and evaluated in the early 1990s. MBCT brought together concepts and approaches from Mindfulness Based Stress Reduction and some from cognitive therapy including approaches developed by Philip Barnard and John Teasdale. Barnard and Teasdale proposed that there was therapeutic value in moving towards a state of mind described as "being": where one is focused in accepting things as they currently are. MBCT aims to train patients to try and "decenter" their thoughts. To accept them as transient and simply occurrences in the mind that will pass. An individual should learn to be more focused on the present rather than concerned about the past or future possibilities. To be able to accept the transient presence of thoughts without attributing undue significance to them.

MBCT was initially developed as a group intervention, provided over eight weeks, and focused not on the treatment of depression but on the prevention of depressive relapses. This makes considerable sense to me: many highly depressed patients really struggle to meaningfully engage in mindfulness practices but may enthusiastically and successfully do so once their mood has improved. Once their concentration, focus, and motivation have at least partially been restored. The use of MBCT in relapse prevention has been supported by a number of clinical trials although it is worthy of note that success is dependent on the degree to which patients engage in mindfulness activities outside of the therapy sessions*.

So, if all these treatments are viable treatment options, where do they fit? Clearly, as we started out discussing, psychotherapeutic approaches have the greatest degree of application in patients with more mild or moderately severe depression or perhaps application in patients with persistent symptoms and a history of trauma and challenging life experiences. Patients who are severely depressed will frequently lack the motivation, concentration, and energy to actively engage in the therapeutic process. Some patients will feel too pessimistic, too hopeless, or worthless to feel there is value in engagement. For others, it will feel just too hard. This will not apply to all patients with more severe depression, however, severity should never be used as an automatic reason to deny patients the opportunity to undertake therapy.

What about the patient who has failed to respond to initial medication treatment as will be the focus of much of this book? The patient whose depression is more challenging to treat? What is the role of therapy in treatment resistant depression?

There have been a number of studies that have tried to answer this. To investigate whether forms of psychotherapy (mostly, but not only,

---

* Parsons, Christine E.; Crane, Catherine; Parsons, Liam J.; Fjorback, Lone Overby; Kuyken, Willem (2017). "Home practice in Mindfulness-Based Cognitive Therapy and Mindfulness-Based Stress Reduction: A systematic review and meta-analysis of participants' mindfulness practice and its association with outcomes". Behavior Research and Therapy. 95: 29–41. doi:10.1016/j.brat.2017.05.004. PMC 5501725. PMID 28527330.

CBT) are helpful in patients that have not responded well to medication. Some of these studies have just included patients who had failed one medication: others have included a more varied, more severe, and more chronic sample of patients. Some directly compared therapy to so called "treatment as usual" (which usually means medication). Most, however, compared psychotherapy *added* to medication to medication alone.

Several recent analyses have found no benefit of therapy over treatment as usual: trying further courses of medication or trying psychotherapy appear to have similar benefits in patients who have initially struggled to get better with medication. However, there does appear to be significant (but modest) value in adding therapy to medication treatment.* If medication alone is not working, it seems better to try a combination of therapy and medication rather than just continuing with the drugs. In sum, therapy is no better or worse than medication used alone but adding therapy to medication may well be better than medication by itself. That, like many but certainly not all conclusions of research, seems fairly obvious. If you have only tried medication so far and are struggling to get better, engaging in psychotherapy as well is a sensible thing to do.

It is also true that the research on psychotherapy has not clearly suggested that any one form of therapy is likely to be better than any other. However, they are also clearly not all "equal." I think trying to distinguish whether any one is better overall, however, is a fairly useless exercise. What clearly matters is what is best for each person. This is not likely to be the same, despite what various proponents of different approaches are likely to propose. Just as one form of medication might theoretically be better suited to a specific type of depression, the choice of therapy is ideally individually tailored. An individual who becomes depressed in the context of recurrent problematic relationships is likely to be a better candidate for interpersonal therapy or brief psychodynamic therapy than

---

* Ijaz S, Davies P, Williams CJ, Kessler D, Lewis G, Wiles N. Psychological therapies for treatment-resistant depression in adults. Cochrane Database of Systematic Reviews 2018, Issue 5. Art. No.: CD010558. DOI: 10.1002/14651858.CD010558.pub2. Van Bronswijk, S., Moopen, N., Beijers, L., Ruhe, H., & Peeters, F. (2019). Effectiveness of psychotherapy for treatment-resistant depression: A meta-analysis and meta-regression. *Psychological Medicine, 49*(3), 366-379. doi:10.1017/S003329171800199X

behavioral activation. Dialectical behavioral therapy or schema therapy are two relatively recently developed therapy approaches that are especially suitable for patients with histories of significant trauma.

How do you navigate these choices? Well, hopefully with the assistance of a therapist, psychiatrist, or even family doctor who has some understanding of your personal needs and circumstances. The starting point really is a comprehensive assessment and formulation: the latter guiding a sensible selection of a therapeutic approach tailored to your individual needs.

However, it pays to do some background research and ask lots of questions. Whilst there are plenty of great clinicians out there who will provide unbiased and sensible advice, the quality, training, and experience of therapists of all sorts varies considerably. There are way too many who provide some generic form of counseling or support when a specific evidence-based treatment approach is called for. There are others who will try and make your issues fit into the way they want to provide treatment, rather than the other way around. Therapy approaches can attract zealots: individuals with a belief in what they are doing that is disproportionate to the evidence that it is useful. It is hard to detect and avoid these people. What is possible, and is appropriate, is to ask lots of questions (see below). If the therapist is reluctant to answer the questions, it should be a red flag and you should seriously consider whether this is going to be the right person for you.

### Questions to Ask a Prospective Therapist

- What type of therapy do you propose?
- Why do you think this is the best approach for me?
- What other approaches do you think would be helpful? Why have you chosen this approach?
- What training/experience do you have with this type of therapy?
- What should I expect? How can it help me?
- Are there side effects or complications? Be very suspicious of anyone who denies any treatment can have negative effects.

I want to end this chapter with a few words about the role of self-help books. There are many bookshelves filled with tomes proposing how to help you overcome depression. As author Mark Mason has written, *"there are approximately 3,102 crappy books out there promising to wave a little wand and sprinkle fairy dust in your ass, and everything will instantly be better."** There are many types of self-help books. Some describe the experiences of individuals who have suffered depression and the ways they have found to live with or overcome its challenges. These are less likely to give you the tools to help you recover, but can be helpful by pointing out useful pathways to take. They can also provide an important sense that you are not alone in your battle with depression.

Others provide more esoteric theories about depression, linking its genesis to spiritual or lifestyle problems. Some are quite explicitly therapeutic in focus: there are books directly describing how to undertake the core tasks of many of the common forms of psychotherapy: there are many books outlining CBT, often with a workbook structure, others on ACT and mindfulness based therapy. Finally, there are books that take a more scientific approach—describing elements of biological theories of depression and how these can be used to understand or overcome depression.

Are these of any value? They certainly can be. They can provide an opportunity for someone with depression to come to an understanding that what they are undergoing is a shared experience, that others have suffered in this way. The sense of aloneness that can come with depression can be profoundly overwhelming and connection with the experiences of others can be extremely valuable. There can also be direct value in using the therapeutic workbooks and guides. Engaging in therapy guided by books is referred to as bibliotherapy. This may be undertaken with or without parallel engagement in more traditional forms of therapy and can be effective for milder forms of depression.

The biggest concern I have with self-help books is the degree to which so many of them propose to have what is effectively a one size fits all solution to depression for everyone. This is clearly unrealistic and can

* https://markmanson.net/5-books-for-dealing-with-anxiety-and-depression

elevate the expectations of patients, provide false hope, and set individuals up for inevitable failure. This is likely to lead to further self-blame, doubt, and hopelessness. With reasonable expectations, however, they can be of value for some patients and families: providing information and a guide to therapeutic engagement that is not confronting and may help open the door to one-on-one therapy.

In summary, some form of psychological treatment or support will be part of the management of any person who is struggling with significant depression. This may vary from highly structured and very specific psychological treatment provided directly as an intervention for depression to something that helps the patient get through whilst they are waiting for other forms of treatment, more typically of a biological nature, to start to work.

# 3

# ANTIDEPRESSANT MEDICATION: THE PROMISE AND THE PROBLEMS

WﾞﾞHEN WE LEFT Steven in Chapter 1, we had come to an understanding that he has depression, a disorder affecting his thinking, his mood, his energy, and motivation. He was clearly substantially impaired by his depression and it was having a profound impact on his ability to work and socialize. When addressing depression from a clinical perspective, there are multiple things to take into account before, or at the same time as, initiating medication.

As has already been discussed, these will include the need to consider the suitability of the patient for engagement in psychotherapy. There are other things that should also be addressed in most, if not all patients. What is the patient's sleep pattern like, and can this be improved? Can they be encouraged to eat a healthier diet? To exercise more? Is there the possibility that they have an underlying medical condition? Are they drinking too much? Using illicit or prescription drugs that could explain things? At a minimum all patients should be educated more about depression, the things that can impact it and the things they can do that might help.

Non-specific treatment approaches that should be considered in all patients with depression:

- Improve sleep patterns by addressing basic sleep hygiene
- Reduce or stop problematic alcohol or drug consumption
- Improve diet
- Engage in regular exercise
- Cessation of smoking

While these are addressed, many patients, as was Steven, will be more interested in antidepressant medication treatment. But what are these so-called antidepressants? Are they really a sensible treatment option? These will be the questions I hope to answer in this chapter.

The core of mainstream biological treatment for depression since the late 1950s has been the use of a series of antidepressant medications. The first antidepressants were very much discovered by chance. Isoniazid was already a relatively old drug by the time doctors first discovered it could help depression: first synthesized in 1912 and more recently recognized as having potential value in the treatment of tuberculosis. In the early 1950s several psychiatrists reported trying to use it therapeutically in the treatment of schizophrenia. It was a publication, in 1953, however, that stimulated interest in its use in depression. Harry Salzer and Max Lurie, two psychiatrists in Cincinnati, reported that year on the treatment of 41 patients with isoniazid—almost all depressed patients seen in a private psychiatric practice.* Twenty one of the patients had received electric shock therapy for previous episodes of depression. However, 28 of the patients improved substantially to isoniazid. Of the remainder, seven subsequently responded to electroshock therapy and five did not. Interestingly, the improvement seen was usually noted within the first

* Salzer, H. M. (1953). Anxiety and Depressive States Treated With Isonicotinyl Hydrazide (Isoniazid). Archives of Neurology And Psychiatry, 70(3), 317. doi:10.1001/archneurpsyc.1953.023203300420

three weeks of therapy, something that was not considered consistent with a spontaneous resolution of depression.

In the same year of this publication, chemists at the pharmaceutical company Hoffmann-La Roche Ltd in the USA synthesized a new compound in their search for novel drugs for the potentially deadly tuberculosis: the creatively named iproniazid. Euphoria and mood change was noted in patients with TB treated with iproniazid and in 1957, its benefits in depressed patients were reported by several New York psychiatrists. This led to a rapid expansion of "off label" use (use of a drug for a non-approved indication)—at least 400,000 patients were reported to receive iproniazid in the twelve months following the initial reports on its use.* Iproniazid did not last long however, it caused liver damage, but its discovery led to the development of a class of antidepressants, the monoamine oxidase inhibitors (MAOI), several of which are still in use today.

At the same time this was all going on, a second drug was also found to have value in the treatment of depression, also pretty much by accident. This drug, imipramine, was being tested as a possible new treatment for schizophrenia, when it was found to have significant antidepressant effects. It is still used today and its discovery triggered the development of a second class of medications for depression: the tricyclic antidepressants (TCAs). By the 1970s amongst others we had imipramine, amitriptyline, trimipramine, clomipramine, nortriptyline and desipramine. At least Pfizer showed some originality in naming their TCA drug doxepin.

The development of the MAOI and TCA antidepressants profoundly changed the treatment of depression and also, as noted in Chapter 1, the way psychiatry saw the cause of depression. However, these drugs were not easy to prescribe and monitor—doses needed to be increased slowly and patients monitored carefully for side effects—and so antidepressant medication therapy remained mostly a specialist activity until the late 1980s. Then, Prozac changed everything. Prozac, or fluoxetine, was first

---

* Vitor Silva Pereira, Vinícius Antonio Hiroaki-Sato Acta Neuropsychiatrica, Volume 30, Issue 6 December 2018, pp. 307-322

synthesized by Eli Lily in the early 1970s in the quest to develop a drug that had quite specific effects in increasing serotonin activity in the brain. Its effects on psychiatric treatment, and popular culture, were unprecedented as it rapidly became a "blockbuster" drug.*

Why did it become popular so quickly? For a start, it was dramatically easier to prescribe than the older antidepressant drugs. Instead of having to slowly increase the drug dose over several weeks, a patient could be started on a therapeutic dose straight away. It was much safer to take, and it was promoted heavily as having a much improved side effect profile.** The side effects of fluoxetine and the other SSRIs that followed were certainly different from the older drugs and if not less common, possibly less severe. Some of the problems that later became apparent with the drug, including sexual dysfunction and increasing suicidal ideation in young patients, were not apparent early on, as we will discuss further, partly due the systematic suppression of relevant medical information from the clinical trials by Eli Lilly.

The ease of prescribing this new class of antidepressants, and an emerging recognition of how common depression was, expanded the treatment of depression from a specialist activity to the domain of general practice, in no doubt facilitated by an extremely effective marketing machine. The use of these drugs exploded, both in sales and cultural impact. Best sellers like *Prozac Nation* and *Listening to Prozac* drew widespread attention. The profits rolled into Eli Lilly, Pfizer and the other companies who developed SSRIs and jumped onto this lucrative bandwagon.

The potency and extent of the marketing that supported the introduction of Prozac, and later other SSRIs, cannot be underestimated in considering the influences supporting its widespread use. As discussed by

* Blockbuster drugs are high selling drugs, often defined as drugs selling more than $1 Billion per year

** The older classes of antidepressants were quite dangerous when taken in overdose and tricyclic antidepressants could cause problems for patients with heart disease. It is questionable whether these new drugs had fewer side effects than the older ones, they certainly had different side effects

Nathan Greenslit and Ted Kaptchuk in 2012,* Prozac was supported by an advertising campaign that especially emphasized its pharmacological selectivity, and by inference, superiority. Marketing campaigns create a veneer of truth; replacing the uncertainty of psychopharmacological science with simple digestible ideas of what causes depression and how this is addressed with impressive precision with "selective" medications.

The development of the SSRIs has now been followed by the introduction of a series of different medications of varying classes and mechanisms of action. SNRIs affect noradrenaline as well as serotonin: these have become a widely prescribed group of drugs. Whereas Eli Lilly was initially focused on selectivity in the development of fluoxetine. The development of SNRIs was a partial reversal, back towards the TCAs and MAOIs, drugs affecting multiple neurochemical pathways. In the case of SNRIs, this was a focus on both serotonin and noradrenaline, the two neurochemicals most widely and consistently implicated in depression.

By affecting two pathways, SNRIs offer a promise of increased efficacy over the more selective SSRIs. However, the inevitable result should be that if you affect two pathways, there is twice the chance of benefit and twice the chance of side effects. The data suggest that there is some truth to this, although the benefits and side effects are clearly not twice as common. SNRIs come with all the side effects of SSRIs, plus some more unique ones of their own such as elevated blood pressure.

Interpreting what we know about comparative efficacy is a challenge. If you look at all the clinical trials conducted that compared drugs of different classes, these have almost universally been paid for and conducted by "big pharma." There is one consistent predictor of which drug will look the best in these trials and it has nothing to do with medication type: it is the company that has sponsored the trial. If the trial is paid for by a company making an SNRI, their solution will look best. If it is a SSRI manufacturer—guess what is going to shine through? Yes, the SSRI of course. This does not necessarily reflect true differences between these drugs but the subtle ways that trials can be manipulated

* Greenslit NP, Kaptchuk TJ. Antidepressants and advertising: psychopharmaceuticals in crisis. *Yale J Biol Med*. 2012;85(1):153–158.

to meet the needs of the sponsoring company. For example, if you want to show that your drug is more effective than a competitor, you might slightly underdose the patients on the competing drug so they do not do as well. Or you might include patients in the trial who have already not responded to the other drug (and hence will be likely to fail with this again) but not patients who have already tried your medication. In contrast, if you want to show that your medication has fewer side effects, you can have a slightly lower dosing schedule.

A great example of these biases comes from the field of schizophrenia. In 2004 a group of authors published an Eli Lilly sponsored study proposing that their antipsychotic drug olanzapine was just as good as an existing medication, clozapine, in the management of patients with so called treatment—resistant schizophrenia.* Clozapine was recognized as the only medication that was effective in the treatment of patients who had not responded to other antipsychotic drugs. Clozapine was substantially under-dosed in this trial compared to the way in which it would commonly be used by psychiatrists. In contrast, olanzapine was used at the higher end of the dosing range. The drugs looked relatively similar in efficacy and this study was used by the Eli Lilly sales team to propose that olanzapine was as an effective intervention an intervention as clozapine in this patient group. However, the equivalence of the drugs in this study was at least in part secondary to the under dosing of the clozapine and unlikely to reflect a true effect.

Coming back to antidepressants, despite the lack of clarity in the studies, there is a reasonable professional consensus that SNRIs are modestly more effective than SSRIs, but at a cost of greater side effects and risks arising from overdose. As such, they tend to be used "second line"—after a first medication has failed to work—in primary practice. They are more commonly used first in specialist psychiatric practice, especially inpatient psychiatry in quite unwell patients, where the need

* Bitter, I., Dossenbach, M. R.., Brook, S., Feldman, P. D., Metcalfe, S., Gagiano, C. A., . . . Breier, A. (2004). *Olanzapine versus clozapine in treatment-resistant or treatment-intolerant schizophrenia. Progress in Neuro-Psychopharmacology and Biological Psychiatry, 28(1), 173–180.* doi: 10.1016/j.pnpbp.2003.09.033

for maximum efficacy is greatest and might outweigh the higher side effect risk.

Beyond the SSRIs and SNRIs (see Table 3.1), the most commonly used medications are a real mixed bag. Bupropion predominately affects dopamine as well as noradrenaline: the dopamine effect makes it relatively unique and as such, worth consideration when patients cannot tolerate or do not respond to serotonin focused medications. Another option for this group is reboxetine: it is selective for the noradrenaline system. Another commonly prescribed drug is mirtazapine. It is unusual. It is also an SSRI—this effect increases serotonin levels—but at the same time it blocks one of the serotonin receptors, stopping serotonin from working in some pathways. The sum effect of this is that it does not have many of the side effects of standard SSRIs. Most usefully, it usually does not cause problematic long-term sexual dysfunction. It is also quite sedating which can also be very useful. There is always a downside, however. In this case it is that a significant percentage of patients will experience problematic weight gain, having to stop the drug.

The TCAs and MAOI that we discussed before, do remain in use but much less commonly than in the 1970s and 80s. There is a somewhat universal agreement that they are more effective than the newer generations of medications but their side effects and danger of serious medical problems being caused by overdose inhibits more widespread use. The impact of practical dosing issues, as mentioned before, cannot be underestimated. The typical starting dose for an TCA such as imipramine is 25 mg at night. The dose is increased every 3-5 days until a dose of at least 150mg is achieved. The drug is unlikely to work for depression at the lower levels which means several weeks of fiddling around before things even really start—and only a proportion of patients will get there due to side effects, especially lowered blood pressure and sedation. Therefore, these drugs remain in the shadows, used by psychiatrist, usually when they have become relatively desperate due to the failure of many other options.

| TABLE 3.1: DIFFERENT TYPES OF COMMON ANTIDEPRESSANTS | | | |
|---|---|---|---|
| **Class of Drug** | **Intended Effect** | **Common Side Effects** | **Other Issues** |
| **Monoamine Oxidase Inhibitors** | Block the MAO enzyme increasing levels of serotonin, noradrenaline, dopamine | Lowered blood pressure, insomnia | Need a restricted diet |
| **Tricyclic Antidepressants** | Block reuptake of serotonin and noradrenaline out of the connection between nerve cells | Lowered blood pressure Sedation Dry eyes, mouth | Need to very slowly increase dose |
| **Selective Serotonin Reuptake Inhibitors** | Block reuptake of serotonin out of the connection between nerve cells | Nausea, dizziness, sexual dysfunction | Changes in personality |
| **Serotonin Noradrenaline Reuptake Inhibitors** | Block reuptake of serotonin and noradrenaline out of the connection between nerve cells | Nausea, dizziness, sexual dysfunction, increased blood pressure, constipation | Discontinuation common with venlafaxine |
| **Norepinephrine and dopamine reuptake inhibitors (NDRIs)** | Block reuptake of dopamine and noradrenaline out of the connection between nerve cells | Agitation, dry mouth, insomnia, headache/migraine | Can cause seizures especially at higher doses |
| **Noradrenaline and specific serotoninergic antidepressants (NASSAs)** | Have varied effects on serotonin and noradrenaline reuptake and receptors | Constipation, dry mouth, weight gain, drowsiness, and sedation | |

Antidepressant use has now become ubiquitous in Western countries. The US National Center for Health Statistics reported in 2017 that 12.7% of the US population aged 12 years or older took antidepressants over the course of a single month.* One in 4 patients had taken these medications for over 10 years and medication use for depression was increasing: from 7.7% of the population in 1999–2002 to 12.7% in

* Pratt L.A., Brody D.J., & Gu Q. Antidepressant use among persons aged 12 and over: United States, 2011–14. NCHS Data Brief, No. 283. Hyattsville, MD: National Center for Health Statistics. 2017.

2011–2014. As early as 2004 there were reports in the UK press of fluoxetine being found in drinking water. And this is all big business: market research firm in 2019 reported that the global antidepressant market would be worth close to $16 billion by 2023.*

If depression is such a common and troubling condition, what is wrong with such a widespread use of antidepressant medications?

One of the main causes of the backlash against widespread antidepressant use was the recognition of an association between the use of SSRIs and increased suicidal ideation as well as potentially other impulsive or violent behaviors. Slowly in the years after Prozac was released it became apparent that some patients, most typically younger ones, would experience increased suicidal thoughts after starting the drug. However, widespread recognition of this risk required a series of legal actions against Eli Lilly, a process that revealed the systematic suppression of information connecting fluoxetine use and suicidality that was apparent in the clinical trials of Prozac.** If this had been openly presented as an issue when Prozac was first released, the use of these drugs would have evolved, perhaps more slowly, but in a manner designed to provide safe guards for patients. At the simplest level, the prescription of Prozac might have remained a little more like it had in other antidepressants for decades.

Historically, psychiatrists were trained to monitor patients closely in the weeks after antidepressants were started. This was in part a necessity due to the need to start older medications quite slowly but also related to the widespread understanding that patients could become more at risk of suicide after medication was commenced. This increased risk was noted to arise from the way in which patients might start to recover from their depression: in some patients, problems with motivation and energy would improve before they experienced a lifting of thoughts of hopelessness and suicide. A more energized patient was more likely to act on troubling suicidal thoughts than one who was too unwell to engage in active suicidal planning. As such, psychiatrists were used to the idea that risk might

---

* https://www.prnewswire.com/news-releases/antidepressant-drugs-market-to-reach-15-98-bn-by-2023-globally-at-2-1-cagr-says-allied-market-research-873540700.html
** https://www.drugwatch.com/ssri/prozac/lawsuits/

increase before it falls as the patient continues to get better. If SSRIs had a specific effect of increasing suicidal tendencies in some patients, this could be addressed with appropriate education and monitoring. However, that would require open information sharing and education of doctors, something that never happened when Prozac was released, much to the eternal shame of the companies and individuals involved.

As it has subsequently become clear over time, the risk associated with SSRIs and suicide appears to be a quite specific one and not just related to changing depressive symptoms as had been seen with antidepressants before this. Specifically, SSRIs raise suicide risk in adolescent and young adult patients. This does not seem to be the case in older depressed patients commenced on these drugs. In my mind, this only increases the culpability of Eli Lilly; given the risk was limited, it could have been targeted with quite specific education and information without compromising the more widespread role out of the drug.

Despite the extremely heavy promotion of SSRIs as drugs with a very limited side effect profile, the real side effect burden of these drugs has become more apparent over time limiting the willingness of many patients to continue their use. The most common initial side effects, like nausea and dizziness, do tend to fade over time in most people. This is a positive contrast with the older drugs such as TCAs and MAOI where most side effects are really not going to diminish if you persist in taking the medication. Other problems are not so easy to deal with. Effects on sexual desire and performance are extremely common. Just as patients are recovering from their depression, which tends to completely deflate sexual desire itself in most patients, they find they have no interest in reengaging sexually with their partner. This does not abate if the offending drug is continued, and it can have a significant impact on relationships. In addition, a recent analysis suggested that long-term SSRI use seems to be associated with a significant increase in risk of stroke and heart disease.*

* Maslej et al. Psychother Psychosom. 2017;86(5):268-282. DOI: 10.1159/000477940. Epub 2017 Sep 14. The Mortality and Myocardial Effects of Antidepressants Are Moderated by Preexisting Cardiovascular Disease: A Meta-Analysis.

Another persistent effect of treatment in some patients is a blunting of emotional experiences. This is often seen as a symptom of depression itself. However, when this is a continued problem in a patient who has otherwise made a comprehensive recovery, its relationship to medication use is usually fairly clear, motivating many patients to want to discontinue therapy. This change in emotional experience is related to another experience described by some patients and first discussed widely in Peter Kramer's book, *Listening to Prozac*. The experience of some is that their medication use has somehow modified important aspects of their personality. This is not always experienced in a negative manner. Kramer describes patients who had a marked lessening of anxiety that they had previously experienced in social situations, increasing their capacity to function socially and at work. Not unsurprisingly, soon the drugs were being marketed for "social anxiety disorder" a condition whose prominence bloomed now that there was a drug to treat it. Some research has suggested that paroxetine, another SSRI, may reduce the personality trait of neuroticism.* Neuroticism, referring in this context to an uncomfortable self-consciousness and emotional vulnerability, was substantially reduced on medication compared to placebo.

Although there may be an upside to the experience of drug related changes in personality, it is clearly not favorably perceived by many patients. Many patients do not like either the subjective sense of an altered relation to the world around them or the basic idea that they are being modified in some way by medication that is meant to just alleviate a troubling condition. These are often strong motivations for patients to stop antidepressant treatment.

Discontinuation is, however, not always easy. There is clearly a risk of the return of depression whenever someone comes off one of these medications. However, there is frequently—perhaps in as many as one in five patients stopping SSRIs and SNRIs—a greater short-term problem: withdrawal effects. Although initially not widely recognized, it is clear

---

* Tang, T., DeRubeis, R., Hollon, S., Amsterdam, J., Shelton, R. and Schalet, B., 2020. Personality Change During Depression Treatment. Arch Gen Psychiatry. 2009 Dec; 66(12): 1322–1330.

that patients can experience marked withdrawal effects when stopping SSRIs and other antidepressants such as the SNRI venlafaxine. There are a variety of symptoms patients experience when stopping these drugs (see below). The most striking one is often described by patients as 'brain zaps'. This is a distressing experience often described of zaps of electricity coming out of their brain or spinal cord. Often this is so strange patients will not spontaneously reveal they are experiencing it due to embarrassment or fear they are "going crazy".

Withdrawal effects tend to be more severe with medications that are short acting, as the effects of these drugs wear off more quickly. Discontinuation can be lessened by a slow reduction and cessation but unfortunately in some patients this just drags out the pain. The possibility of experiencing discontinuation symptoms is not the same as saying these drugs are addictive. Addiction usually implies a variety of characteristics including escalating use over time and drug seeking behavior as well as withdrawal. By this definition, SSRIs, for all their faults, are not truly addictive. However, discontinuation can be extremely uncomfortable and a strong disincentive to try a second or third medication.

### Distinguishing Withdrawal from Recurrence of Depression

This can be extremely difficult for some patients. Illness recurrence is usually associated with low mood and worsening negative thoughts whereas withdrawal is more typically characterized by increased anxiety and physical symptoms.

Withdrawal symptoms with common antidepressants

- Increased anxiety, agitation, restlessness
- Headaches, dizziness, light-headedness
- Racing heart, sweatiness, nausea
- Brain zaps

All of these are important limitations, but there is another equally essential concern about modern antidepressant drugs: that they are just not that effective. Since the first marketing of Prozac, antidepressants have been persistently presented as a simple and effective solution for depression. This has in part been the message of effective drug marketing and in part the widespread message of public health campaigns designed to lessen stigma around depression and increase access to care. As laudable and important as the latter have been, they often present a simple message: come forward and get diagnosed as treatment is simple and effective. Whether it is medication or psychological interventions, this message is far from the truth.

What do we know about the effectiveness of antidepressants and why are there concerns about this? The vast majority of this knowledge about medication effectiveness comes from the clinical trials evaluating the use of these drugs, sponsored and conducted by the companies responsible for their production, and who will exploit their commercial potential. Clinical trials of new drugs run in phases. In phase 1, limited doses are given to healthy volunteers, to make sure they seem safe, to understand how they are processed by the body and to come to an initial understanding of the right sort of doses to test in patients. In phase 2, increasingly large groups of patients receive the new drug, to establish whether it seems to work and at what dose. Phase 3 is the final hurdle. One, or usually multiple, large, randomized trials where hundreds (or thousands) of patients in many different research centers and clinics receive the drug or a placebo. These trials are usually "double-blind": the patient and their doctor and the person evaluating how effective the drug is, are not allowed to know if they are receiving the real or fake pill.

The Food and Drug Administration (FDA) first seriously began to regulate drug availability in 1938. However, until 1962, drug manufacturers were only required to demonstrate that their products were safe. In response to concerns about inaccurate marketing and precipitated by the disastrous birth defects resulting from the use of thalidomide, the requirement for proof of drug effectiveness was introduced in the 1962 Kefauver-Harris Drug Amendments and the 1963 investigational drug regulations that followed. In the years following the introduction of these rules, the FDA also faced the challenging task of assessing the status of drugs approved and marketed prior to 1962. Their Director of the Bureau of Medicine, Doctor Herbert Ley, led the development of evidence rules whereby companies were required to produce data supporting efficacy based on "well controlled" clinical trials. The rules also specified that positive data be produced from a minimum of two clinical trials.*

This has remained the standard for new drug approval submissions over time. Of note, the standard is that the drug be effective in 2 trials. This could be 2 out of 2 trials, or possibly 2 out of 6 or 2 out of 10. In other words, there could be more trials that showed no benefit of treatment than showed that the drug worked: all they needed were 2 "positive" studies. Even when the rules were changed so that companies were required to register all trials with the FDA, both positive and negative, very few of the negative studies were actually published in professional journals and became publicly available.

How bad was this? Pretty bad! An analysis in 2008 showed that all but one of the positive antidepressant studies conducted before that time were published: there was no hesitation to bring the good news to the world.** However, the vast majority of negative studies were not published or were published with misleading results. Overall, only 51% of trials actually showed a benefit from the drugs. However, 94% of the published trials showed a positive benefit. A doctor, or anyone else reading these studies to appraise whether these drugs were effective, would get an overwhelmingly positive impression. The consequences of this were not trivial. When a new drug was released, the marketing people would bring doctors copies of the 2 positive studies—"look, our drug works great." No one was the wiser as to whether these trials were the exceptions or the rule.

---

* "FDA and Clinical Drug Trials: A Short History," in A Quick Guide to Clinical Trials, Madhu Davies and Faiz Kerimani, eds. (Washington: Bioplan, Inc.: 2008), pp. 25-55.
** Selective Publication of Antidepressant Trials and Its Influence on Apparent Efficacy. Erick H. Turner, M.D., Annette M. Matthews, M.D., Eftihia Linardatos, B.S., Robert A. Tell, L.C.S.W., and Robert Rosenthal, Ph.D. N Engl J Med 2008;358:252-60.

An increasing awareness of these issues in the 2000s motivated researchers to question whether the body of existing studies, published or not, really supported whether antidepressants—especially SSRIs—work. In 2002, Irving Kirsch from the University of Hull in the UK obtained data from all the trials of SSRI medications conducted to that time and subjected these to a process called meta-analysis. Meta-analysis is a statistical approach that combines the effects seen across multiple clinical trials and is widely regarded as one of the most important ways to judge whether a treatment is truly effective. The results of this study took many people by surprise, gathered much attention and sparked intense debate.

When compared to placebo (fake pills), the SSRIs did not look all that good. The analysis showed that active drugs produced only a 1.8-point greater reduction on average than placebo pills on the Hamilton Rating Scale of Depression (HRSD). The HRSD is a questionnaire used by researchers or doctors to measure depression severity (see box on the next page). The National Institute for Clinical Excellence (NICE) in the UK regards a 3-point difference between active drug and placebo, the minimum standard for a clinically meaningful difference: antidepressants in this analysis did not come close to this. The meaning of this study, and similar ones, have been intensely debated with some proposing that the data fundamentally disputes the idea that modern antidepressant medications are effective at all. Other analyses have suggested that anti-depressants are only more effective in more severely depressed patients (who are often under-represented in clinical trials; see box).* Whether these studies truly deny the efficacy of these medications is not really of concern here. What matters is that even if the data supports efficacy, the strength of the benefits of these medications is really limited.

* Kirsch I, Deacon BJ, Huedo-Medina TB, Scoboria A, Moore TJ, Johnson BT: Initial severity and antidepressant benefits: a meta-analysis of data submitted to the Food and Drug Administration. PLoS Med. 2008, 5 (2): e45 10.1371/journal.pmed.0050045

## How are the Benefits of Depression Treatments Established in Clinical Trials?

Clinical trials typically compare the improvements in depression produced by a new medication (or other type of therapy) to that seen with a fake treatment – in the case of medication, a sugar pill or placebo. There are, however, no simple tests to ascertain whether depression has gone away – there is no form of brain scanning that can distinguish the brain of a patient with depression from one without with sufficient accuracy to be clinically useful. Therefore, clinical trials use questionnaires to try and reliably assess the severity of depression. These typically have between 10 and 25 questions addressing different aspects of the symptoms of depression. A score (usually on a scale of 0-4 or 0-5) is allocated to each question. For example, on a question about sleep disturbance, a 5 might indicate the patient has trouble sleeping every night or sleeps less than 3 hours whereas a 0 indicates normal sleep.

Two types of instruments are used—ones that are completed by a trained rater who asks the patient questions and ones directly completed by patients. Examples of the former include the Hamilton Depression Rating Scale, the Montgomery and Asberg Depression Rating Scale, and the Inventory of Depressive Symptoms. The Beck Depression Inventory is the most well-known example of the latter.

As well as tools assessing the severity of depression, clinical trials will usually include other measures to evaluate side effects, overall functioning and quality of life. Quality of life tools generally assess the satisfaction an individual feels about different aspects of their life as well as their capacity to function in different roles.

There is another highly influential study that has provided valuable information as to what patients can expect with antidepressant medication. The STAR*D study was a large trial funded independently of the pharmaceutical industry by the National Institute for Mental Health in the US. In this trial, 2,876 patients with an episode of depression were commenced on the SSRI medication citalopram. If they failed to respond adequately to this, they were randomized to one of several medication alternatives and the process was repeated through a total of 4 stages.

Of note, this study did not involve a placebo control: typically studies without a placebo group tend to show greater effects of medication. Only 28% of patients remitted (had full recovery) with the initial trial of medication and remission rates fell progressively across each level of treatment. For example, patients having not responded to two medications then only had a less than 15% chance of responding to the next option. After progressing through all of the various stages of treatment, one third of patients had failed to achieve a meaningful clinical benefit. Patients who had failed to respond to the first or second medication had a very low rate of treatment success and only one in 20 patients who failed the initial two medications subsequently got better and remained well after a year.

## How Well Do Clinical Trials Do in Assessing the Value of Antidepressant Medications?

Whether standard clinical trial methods have under-estimated, or over-estimated, antidepressant effects have been the focus of considerable concern. Clinical trials historically have been conducted in academic medical centers. These have historically been hospital based and may not necessarily service a population of patients that is the same as that seen in more widespread community health settings. This could lead to trials not really testing new drugs in a group of patients like the majority of those who will receive these drugs after they are marketed. These studies are said not to be "representative" of the patients who will take the medication in the future. At times, these centers have also been criticized for potentially cycling a small population of patients with long term illness through multiple trials over time.

Over time an industry of private trial centers has developed which exist exclusively to conduct clinical trials. These centers do not provide clinical service and as such rely on advertising to recruit patients into clinical trials. These patients may be of lesser severity than those typically treated in clinical services and are certainly different. If the patients are generally less severe than 'real world' clinical patients, this potentially will lead to trials under-estimating clinical effects if the drugs are more effective in more severely unwell patients.

Patients who have a milder illness are also more likely to experience a placebo response. This is when a patient gets better when taking the fake pill against which the new drug is being tested. Overall, rates of patients responding to placebo in trials of antidepressant medications are often around 3 or 4 in every 10 patients. This is especially the case for patients with less severe depression (where some patients might just get better spontaneously, without any active treatment). The consequence is that the real medication must work much better than this for it to be seen to be effective in a trial.

There are other concerns as well. Commercial trial centers, as well as academic ones, are likely to have strong financial incentives to include patients. Staff assessing patients may also have unconscious biases that increases their chance of including patients who are not quite sick enough to meet the criteria for the study. They may not want to disappoint patients who come along interested in trial participation (especially when there are financial incentives to take part) and may be financially motivated to recruit quickly themselves. This may all lead to subtle "up-scoring" of patients on depression severity scales to ensure they fit the severity criteria for inclusion in the studies. For example, staff scoring patients' depression severity may err on the side of a 5 instead of a 4, a 3 instead of a 2. After patients are included in a trial, their depression severity scores are likely to revert to a lower level better reflecting the true severity of their illness, just reflecting their real level of symptoms, not real improvement. This will make both the groups of patients taking the active drug and those taking the placebo look like they are improving. An increase in the placebo response in this way is really problematic as it makes it very difficult for a trial to show a meaningful benefit of the active drug if the placebo treated patients do too well.

These studies, in summary, cast serious doubt on the degree of overall short-term efficacy of medication therapy and are likely to give many patients cause to rethink treatment choices, especially given some of the previously documented downsides of this form of treatment. But what about the long-term?

Concerns have also been raised as to the long-term impact of antidepressant prescribing on the course of depression. Roger Whitaker, in *Anatomy of an Epidemic* published in 2010, argued the case that although antidepressants may work in the short-term, they induce changes in the brains of patients that result in an increased likelihood of future relapse and worse overall outcomes. Whitaker quotes Amy Upham from 2009 saying "*With psychiatric medications, you solve one problem for a period of time, but the next thing you know you end up with two problems. The treatment turns a period of crisis into a chronic mental illness.*"

One possibility is that increasing serotonin levels above normal with an SSRI—remembering that serotonin levels were probably not low in the first place—will in some cases reset whatever mechanism underlies an individual patient's depression in the short term. However, neural systems will adapt to this pharmacologically induced increase in a manner that heightens future vulnerability to depression: perhaps by decreasing the receptors for serotonin to dampen down the overactive system or by altering serotonin production.

It is worth noting that most antidepressants have been evaluated in follow-up studies showing that their use, typically over 12 months, reduces illness relapse. Over this time frame, they seem to keep more people well than are kept well by placebo tablets. Whitaker is arguing, however, that over a longer time, the situation is potentially the opposite. The reality is that we lack the research to meaningfully answer the question of the impact of antidepressants on long-term outcomes. There are no randomized controlled trials that extend over decades. There are also not going to be any of these in the foreseeable future. Ethics committees and patients are not going to agree to years of potential placebo treatment.

Whitaker's premise is based, in part, on comparisons of outcomes for depression from the pre-medication era to the present. So many other factors have changed, however, in how we diagnose and treat depression that this is by no means definitive evidence. For example, even the basic concepts of what is depression and the mechanism of diagnosis have altered unrecognizably in the last 50 years. In the pre-medication era, there were really no standardized systems for psychiatric diagnosis. The diagnostic practice was determined by localized training and experience. The likelihood of receiving a specific diagnosis, for example of schizophrenia or bipolar disorder, differed markedly between countries. The advent of the Diagnostic and Statistical Manual (DSM) in its various modern forms since the 1980s has provided a standardized tool kit to maximize the chance of consistent diagnostic practice. The spread of antidepressant prescribing into general practice in particular also indicates that we are treating a vastly expanded group of patients now than were receiving psychiatric treatment in the era of long-term incarceration in asylums. All of these factors will have affected the outcomes of depression over time. How much so, and how much of an influence antidepressants have had on long-term depression outcomes, remains quite unclear.

So where does that leave us? Is it reasonable to put faith in the use of antidepressant medications in the management of substantial depression? Well, there are patients who will be helped by these medications, and probably many more who will be helped by a decent dose of the placebo effect. Although side effects are common, many patients do tolerate these medications quite well and fortunately, some respond to treatment, at best achieving full recovery of the episode of depression they are experiencing.

Unfortunately, the picture is not so rosy for many more. Some individuals will not respond at all. Others will get better but experience a return of their symptoms. Sometimes this is after a long interval, sometimes only after a very brief period of time. Frequently patients experience "poop out," a repeated short-lived benefit from medication: patients get an early, sometimes substantial improvement. However, this goes away quickly. They start another medication, and the cycle starts again. This pattern of repeated short-lived responses to medication and marked relapse of symptoms can go on for many years and the patient continues to struggle to find a meaningful therapeutic strategy.

If this all sounds a little grim, and perhaps not the rosy picture one might get from pharmaceutical advertising, it is the reality for many patients with depression. Antidepressant medications are not the magic bullets we would like them to be. In the following chapters we will explore some of the alternatives and where these might fit in.

# 4

# MOVING BEYOND MEDICATION

A FEW YEARS AGO, I saw a middle-aged woman in her early 40s, let's call her Anne. Anne was born the third child of 4 in a relatively well-off upper middle class family. Her father worked as a banking executive. Her mother was a teacher who had stopped working after her second child was born to raise her children. Anne had a peaceful and happy early life: she was very close to her mother and older sister, but perhaps less so with her father who worked long hours. She experienced no significant traumas in childhood, had a good range of friends, and did well at school. After school she attended university and became a teacher like her mother. In the third year of university she experienced what sounded in retrospect like an episode of depression triggered by the breakdown of a romantic relationship. She saw a university counselor for a few months and eventually her mood improved. She married at age 28 and had 2 children in her early 30s.

At age 38 she experienced what this time was very clearly an episode of major depressive disorder. There was no major precipitant, but she had been worried for a while about her husband who was having some issues at work, and about her youngest child, a boy, who was having some mild learning issues. After a few weeks of rapidly worsening mood, she saw her family doctor who referred her to a psychologist and commenced her on the SSRI drug citalopram. She took 20mg a day of this for about 2½ months, and saw her psychologist weekly, but saw no improvement at all. She remained flat, unmotivated, miserable, and lethargic. After this time her doctor referred her to a psychiatrist and switched the citalopram to another SSRI, sertraline, at 50mg a day, a quite low dose. She stayed on this for the 2 months it took to get an appointment with the psychiatrist who then progressively increased the sertraline over several weeks to 200mg per day. Again, without any benefit.

After another month, and with Anne in a state of increasing desperation, the sertraline was switched to an SNRI, venlafaxine, and a low dose of the antipsychotic quetiapine was also started, she was told it was to help with her sleep. Again, no change. The venlafaxine was increased to 150mg but not higher as she developed quite severe headaches and it was eventually switched to another SSRI, this time fluoxetine. She was taking the fluoxetine two months later when she came to see me for a second opinion, still profoundly depressed, many months after first presenting for treatment.

Anne's story is notable, not in the rarity of her presentation, but because of how common it is. Many, many patients with depression go on harrowing journeys like hers. They cycle through medication after medication, often seeing doctor after doctor, psychologist after psychologist. Some spend time in hospital, most do not. All suffer, as do their loved ones. The pattern of her treatment is also fairly common; many patients will have trials of multiple medications, but they are often similar in type. In Anne's case, she had experienced trials of four SSRI's, especially given that the venlafaxine dose was not increased over 150mg (at low dose venlafaxine is effectively an SSRI, its effects on noradrenaline only kick in at higher doses), along with a low dose of an antipsychotic: this may have helped her sleep but was never going to fix her depression. What other options did she have? What could or should have been done differently? We will start to address these questions in this chapter.

One factor that is worthy of consideration before we progress, concerns timing. An important feature of the process of trying medications for depression is that this process should not be overly extended in time. It is generally believed that if an antidepressant is not working at all, like for Anne, the treatment period should definitely be no more than six to eight weeks. In fact, if you are going to get better with one of these drugs it is likely you will notice something in the first three weeks. The recommendations for a reasonable medication trial are coming down.

They used to be several months, but now many authorities say three weeks at a good dose is enough.

Anne's therapy was not this prompt at all. However, it was not nearly as prolonged as that experienced by many patients. For many, trials of individual medications can drag on for months and months, just prolonging suffering unnecessarily. Dithering inaction equals bad treatment. Patients and their carers need encouragement to be strong advocates for their care. To not tolerate indecision, to ask difficult questions, and if necessary to seek out new help or advice.

Unfortunately, like Anne, many millions of patients are faced with the challenge of what to do once an antidepressant medication, or several, has failed to work. They might have been given considerable hope that the medication was going to be the solution. Despite the inherent pessimism that comes with being depressed, they may have clung to this hope, along with the pharmaceuticals, and at best managed to get by without a swag of side effects. At worst, they got side effects and withdrawal symptoms to boot. Now what?

Before directly considering whether an individual patient should be exploring alternative treatments, it is always important to take a step back and reassess whether pursuing these or any further medication treatments really makes any sense. If a patient has failed to respond to one or more medication treatments, this should at least prompt a reconsideration as to whether this was a sensible thing to be doing in the first place.

It may not have been. The question needs to be asked. *Were you really suffering from depression? Was it a type of depression that medication may work for?* It is possible that the diagnosis itself was wrong and the medication did not work because depression was not really the problem. There are many things that may have been confused with depression and clarifying the diagnosis is critical before one goes farther with treatment.

First, there might be a mental health condition, just not depression. As discussed earlier, one of the first conditions that should be considered in patients with changes in mood is bipolar disorder, the modern name for manic depression. As a reminder, bipolar disorder is a condition where patients do experience periods of depression, and these are almost exactly the same in presentation as episodes of depression experienced by patients who do not have bipolar disorder. However, these patients, at some point in time, will also go through one or more "manic" episodes. These are also considered episodes of mood change but are very different, and commonly seen as the opposite "pole" of depression. Instead of feeling excessively sad, when manic patients experience persistently, seemingly excessively, good moods. They can be persistently euphoric, even in the light of major problems. However, the person's mood can also change rapidly, bounce from low to high in seconds or the person might have periods of significant agitation or anger.

Mania, like depression, also results in a range of symptoms in addition to an altered mood. Patients usually have lots of energy and are sped up, their thoughts are quick and speech rapid. They do not need to sleep and want to take on lots of projects or activities. Whether they can follow through with these tends to depend on how bad the mania is. More severely unwell patients tend to be quite scattered and jump from thing to thing, not achieving much. Manic patients also take risks and are disinhibited. They commonly will overspend, gamble, or be sexually promiscuous whilst unwell.

Although patients with bipolar disorder, when depressed, have the same depressive symptoms as non-bipolar depressed individuals, they do not tend to do well with antidepressant medication—the medications frequently don't help—and they can even trigger an episode of mania. Undiagnosed bipolar disorder may well be the underlying cause for a lack of medication response. Patients with depression should always be carefully questioned to establish if they have ever experienced an episode of mania in the past. If there is any suggestion that this is the case, the medication management is likely to be quite different.

A so called "adjustment disorder" or "stress response syndrome" is another mental health condition that may have been incorrectly diagnosed as depression. An adjustment disorder is a condition that is directly the result of some significant trauma or life stress. Patients will often experience a mixture of anxiety and depressive symptoms, but the expectation is that these will be less persistent than when seen in an episode of depression, more directly linked to life events, and likely to resolve over time, especially as the stressor is resolved. The treatment of a stress related disorder is predominately psychological, and the use of antidepressant medication is likely to be both ineffective and distracting from appropriate therapy.

Another critical condition to detect that may mimic a presentation of depression is drug or alcohol dependence. Alcohol and many other drugs, including opiates (whether taken on prescription or illegally), are "depressant" drugs. They can produce significant depressive symptoms when taken regularly for extended periods of time. Treating someone who has developed depressive symptoms during a lengthy period of heavy drinking, without changing the drinking pattern at the same time, is likely to be pointless. As well as drugs used for recreational purposes, there are also other prescription drugs that can produce depressive symptoms, so clearly all of the medications and substances being taken by someone presenting with depression need to be clearly explored.

As well as drugs, there are physical ailments that can produce depressive symptoms themselves. For example, when patients have low levels of a substance called thyroid hormone being produced in their body, they can experience both physical slowing down and a profoundly lowered mood. Other imbalances in substances in the body or the failure of various organs can produce symptoms that can be confused with depression. A thorough revaluation of a patient's physical state is warranted if they are not responding to medication, especially if these causes were not thoroughly excluded prior to the commencement of treatment in the first place.

There is also the possibility that a patient has not responded to medication because they have another disorder instead of depression, a poor response to treatment often occurs because the patient has another disorder *as well as* depression. The co-occurrence of two conditions is referred to as "co-morbidity". These co-morbid conditions can be mental or physical, a mixture of both, or involve co-morbid drug or alcohol abuse. Mental health conditions that commonly co-occur with depression include things such as post-traumatic stress disorder, anorexia, and obsessive-compulsive disorder. There are even high rates of depression in patients with things like Alzheimer's disease and autism. Ignoring the co-morbid condition and expecting depression to just respond to antidepressant medication is often wishful thinking.

There is one final consideration in reviewing why a patient may not be getting better: was the dose taken enough? The dose required to get a therapeutic effect with most antidepressants is well established and so this question is not usually complicated to answer. For the SSRIs, the starting dose—for example 20mg of fluoxetine or citalopram—is a therapeutic dose and enough for most patients who will benefit from these drugs. For most of the tricyclic antidepressants, it is at least 150mg a day, a fair bit more than the 25mg that patients get started on and patients frequently don't tolerate a high enough dose to allow one of these drugs to work. If a patient has taken a therapeutic dose for a good enough period of time, a trickier question is whether it is worthwhile to try an even higher dose.

The answer to this, "it depends," is not all that helpful. It is mostly determined by the type of medication the patient has been taking. For SSRIs, there is not a lot of evidence that increasing above the standard dose is likely to be of much value in the treatment of depression (although very importantly, higher doses are usually necessary when SSRIs are used in anxiety disorders and obsessive-compulsive disorder; see below). A patient might respond to an SNRI like venlafaxine at a higher dose due to the specific mechanism of action of this medication. For the older medications like the tricyclic antidepressants, there does seem to be a greater degree of response at higher doses: some patients respond at 150mg/day but others might need 200mg or even 300mg.

| Medication | Standard Dose | Higher Dose | High Dose (for OCD) |
|------------|---------------|-------------|---------------------|
| Fluoxetine | 20mg | 40mg | 60-100mg |
| Paroxetine | 20mg | 40mg | 60-100mg |
| Sertraline | 100mg | 200mg | 300mg |
| Fluvoxamine | 100mg | 200mg | 400mg |
| Citalopram | 20mg | 40mg | 60mg* |
| Escitalopram | 10mg | 20mg | 40mg* |

Standard doses for the SSRI antidepressants, along with the higher doses sometimes tried in depression, and the highest doses most commonly used in the treatment of OCD.
*There are some safety issues with higher doses of these medications.

Therefore, it tends to become a very individual decision. If I had been managing Anne earlier on, I would probably have tried one of the SSRIs at a higher dose, if she was not experiencing side effects, but only for a short time, perhaps two–three weeks. I would see this as a reasonable balance of giving it a try but not wanting to drag things out too long.

So, once all the issues that have been described over the last few pages have been addressed, once the diagnosis is confirmed and intent made to go ahead with medication as a primary option, what are the possibilities when a patient has not responded to initial antidepressant medication treatment? This is often the point at which a family doctor might consider referral to a psychiatrist. The options will include psychological treatments (as discussed in a previous chapter), switching to a second antidepressant, continuing the first and adding a second antidepressant or adding what is often called an "augmentation agent" to the initial antidepressant medication.

Switching from one antidepressant to another is the most common approach when medication 1 has not worked. Many doctors will switch from medication 1 to 2, then from 2 to 3, 3 to 4 . . . for many medication trials whereas other psychiatrists are much more inclined to try combinations of antidepressants and augmentation approaches. Who is right? Before we answer that, let's explore each option a little more.

Switching often seems to make the most obvious sense. If medication 1 is not working, get rid of it and start again. This would especially seem to make sense if medication 1 has caused side effects and if there is no response to it whatsoever. In switching medications, the prescribing doctor is hopefully considering carefully what medication to select next. If, as commonly done, an SSRI has been prescribed initially, the second medication should be something with a different mechanism of action: for example, an SNRI or perhaps bupropion. There is much less sense in trying multiple SSRIs, one after another, as Anne did. Even though these are a little different from each other in subtle ways, they are much more the same than they are different.

Trying something that differs to a greater degree makes much more sense. Venlafaxine is a common second choice but one which should only be undertaken after careful consideration. This is nominally an SNRI so offers a contrast to an initial SSRI. However, this can be misleading. Venlafaxine is only effectively an SNRI when taken at high doses which some doctors may not be comfortable prescribing, and which may produce unacceptable side effects. At lower doses it acts very much as an SSRI: its chemistry is such that it effects serotonin at low doses and its effects on noradrenaline only kick in as the dose is raised above 150mg per day. It is also a medication that can produce some of the worst withdrawal symptoms, especially if the patient is stopping from a high dose. Therefore, before switching from an SSRI to venlafaxine, patients should be warned about these issues and other options considered.

There are three general strategies used by doctors when recommending a switch between antidepressants. In the first, the initial medication is weaned whilst the other one is simultaneously commenced, and the dose increased. There will be an intent to have the second drug up to a therapeutic dose before or at the time the first drug is stopped. This can help with limiting withdrawal symptoms in some patients but usually only if the two medications overlap in how they work. For example, starting a second SSRI will often prevent or limit withdrawal effects from an initial SSRI. However, as described already, if an SSRI has not worked, starting another may not be the best option. A doctor might still sensibly choose to switch from one SSRI to another if the first drug is being stopped for other reasons—such as a side effect or to switch to fluoxetine to help with withdrawal—but this makes less sense if a failure to response to the first SSRI is the reason for stopping.

The second switching method is to start medication 2 and increase this right up to full-dose before any reduction is made of the dose of the first medication. A doctor might be keen to recommend this if there has been some benefit from the first medication, especially in relieving suicidal ideation. The hope is that the second medication starts to work before the first one is stopped so the patient does not worsen in mood, perhaps becoming more suicidal.

## Coping with Antidepressant Withdrawal

Medication withdrawal can cause highly distressing and disabling symptoms. Fortunately, not all patients will experience this. Most patients will want or need to start a new medication quite quickly so it is sensible to try and reduce and stop rapidly at first. If withdrawal symptoms occur, the original dose can be re-started and a much slower reduction commenced. If withdrawal has been experienced coming off this or another medication, the best approach will to be reduce the dose of medication slowly and in the smallest steps possible: the lower the dose, often the slower and smaller the reductions may need to be.

There are some alternatives to completely withdrawing from one medication before starting a new one. Some antidepressants can be taken at the same time as so it might be possible to start medication 2 before stopping medication 1: the effects of the second medication may limit the withdrawal effects of the first. This cannot be done safely with all antidepressants though.

Another alternative for patients stopping some SSRIs is to switch straight from the first SSRI to the SSRI drug fluoxetine and then withdraw from this. Fluoxetine, unlike the other SSRIs, is processed in the body quite slowly. Once you stop it, fluoxetine can be detected in the body for up to 4 weeks. The amount of fluoxetine in the body slowly falls over time. Withdrawal is much less common than with other SSRIs or SNRIs whose effects wear off very quickly.

In the third approach, the initial medication is completely withdrawn prior to commencing the second drug. This approach is "cleaner": it comes with no, or much less risk of interactions between the two drugs, especially if enough of a time gap is allowed between stopping the first and starting the second. Fortunately, for most medications this can be quite quick: there is not much left of most antidepressants in the body after only a few days.

There are a few important, but less common, exceptions. When the old fashion MAOI drugs are stopped, not much else can be started for two weeks. The drugs act by tightly attaching themselves to an enzyme in the brain called monoamine oxidase. This enzyme breaks down brain chemicals like serotonin, noradrenaline, and dopamine. It works to knock out this enzyme, increasing the levels of these neurotransmitters. It does a very thorough job of this. In fact, its effects are irreversible: once it gets to the enzyme, the enzyme will never functionally work again. Therefore, when the drug is stopped, its effects only wear off when the body makes enough new enzyme to replace what has been knocked out: this takes the body several weeks to do. Because its effects are so strong, it is usually not a good idea to combine an MAOI with another antidepressant. The MAOI usually needs to be stopped and 2 weeks allowed to pass before the next medication can start.

Fluoxetine also has prolonged effects, in this case because it hangs around in the body for up to four weeks. This has a major advantage in patients liable to withdrawal effects as it fades away very slowly. The lasting action can also be helpful when it is being taken by people (admit it, most of us are like this!) who struggle to take medication regularly. If you miss a dose of some of the shorter acting medications, for example venlafaxine or the SSRI paroxetine, you can actually get some withdrawal effects even within 24 hours. Perhaps even worse in the long-term, the beneficial effects of the medication might be undermined if the dose in your blood goes up and down a lot with missed doses. Neither of these are an issue with fluoxetine; there is little change in levels of this in the blood if a dose is missed. However, the longer lasting effects create the same problem when switching as those seen with MAOIs. You have to wait even longer, a full four weeks if the new drug might interact badly with the old.

As I am sure you have gotten the impression, the choice of which strategy to adopt really needs to be determined by a doctor trying to balance as many of these concerns as possible. The first two strategies, especially the second, tend to be recommended when patients have had a partial response to initial therapy: the second medication is commenced prior to the withdrawal of the second, hopefully preventing illness deterioration. However, these "cross-titration" approaches do come at a higher risk of interactions and side effects. Strategy 3 is preferable in the situation of complete non-response. The first medication can be withdrawn as rapidly as possible and new treatment initiated without risk of drug interactions or confusion about the source of emergent side effects.

The first situation, choosing what to do with a patient who has made a partial response, is a common and challenging issue. It is not uncommon at all for patients to improve a little on an antidepressant: sometimes the medication might lessen suicidal thoughts or just lift the veil of darkness a little. However, even if the dose is increased and the medication continued for weeks on end, real improvement remains elusive. In this case, switching comes at an obvious cost. Stopping treatment to switch will most likely see these gains lost. Worsening suicidal ideation, perhaps coupled with withdrawal symptoms, will be very unpleasant and possibly dangerous. When this is the case, adding a second therapy as an alternative to switching might make more sense. This could be a second antidepressant or possibly a so-called "augmentation agent" (see below).

### A Brief Word on Language

The use of a second medication added to an antidepressant is often described as "augmentation" or "adjuvant" therapy. Augmentation implies that drug 2 somehow boosts the effects of drug 1—there is little evidence that this is the case with any of the treatments we will discuss. Adjuvant treatment refers to a second, independent, treatment effect: this seems to be the case with the add on therapies that will be discussed here. There might be additional benefits of two drugs over one but they are not combining in a way such that the whole is greater than the sum of the parts.

The use of two or more antidepressants at the same time is a controversial practice in the treatment of depression. Some psychiatrists will go as far as to start two medications at the same time whilst others deem this practice unjustified and potentially harmful. Two medications equal two times the side effects plus potential problems from interactions between the two drugs. One medication can also affect how the body metabolizes the other, changing its effects on the body. The positive side of this would be if there was clear evidence of an advantage of two antidepressants compared to one. Clinical trials have explored this: some saying there is, some not. For now, the value of this approach, certainly as a routine, remains a source of debate.

Combination treatment of this sort is less controversial when used in patients who have not responded to single antidepressant trials (compared to when they are combined in a more routine way). This would more typically be considered after a few medications alone have been unsuccessfully tried, and perhaps even more so when one has produced some limited benefits that you do not want to give up by switching. In reality, any practice is more easily justified when patients are not getting better with more standard approaches.

Regardless of the rationale, there are some medication combinations that are safer than others, and some combinations that make more logical sense. It is generally risky to combine medications with an MAOI (but not all). This can result in a dangerous "serotonin syndrome." It is often problematic to do so with a tricyclic antidepressant: other medications can increase the side effects of this class of medication. SSRIs can be combined with several other medications although it does not really make any sense to combine an SSRI with an SNRI as the SNRI is going to be affecting the serotonin system in pretty much the same way as the SSRI.

One of the more logical antidepressant combinations is an SSRI combined with a noradrenaline reuptake inhibitor (reboxetine is the only one of these commonly available). This effectively produces a drug response similar to that achieved with an SNRI (effects on serotonin and noradrenaline) but where the effects on serotonin and noradrenaline can be adjusted separately by manipulating the dose of one or other of the drugs. In a similar way, an SSRI can be combined with bupropion which affects noradrenaline and dopamine in a manner complementary to the effects of the SSRI on serotonin. This combination seems safe, and the bupropion has even been reported to reduce the sexual side effects seen with SSRIs.* Adding mirtazapine to a SSRI or SNRI is a very common practice. This also can reduce sexual dysfunction as well as improve sleep. Mirtazapine can increase appetite: this can be of benefit in patients struggling to maintain an adequate diet but can also be a real problem for some patients. The combination of mirtazapine and the SNRI venlafaxine has attracted the name "California Rocket Fuel" reflecting both its popularity and a fairly widespread belief in the potency of this combination. Reflecting on my comments about combinations in general, the evidence for this is not consistent and there is clearly a side effect cost of combining these two drugs. It is not something I prescribe on a routine basis or recommend doing so but it may have a role in patients not responding to single medication treatment.

Combination therapy might make more sense in patients not responding to trials of single medications, but does it actually work? The research exploring this is not conclusive. Studies have examined the initiation of 2 antidepressants comparing this to just one and adding a second medication in non-responders to initial therapy, usually with an SSRI. Unfortunately, the results of these studies have been contradictory, not resolving the issue and resulting in considerable diversity of how psychiatrists' practice.

### What is Serotonin Syndrome?

Serotonin syndrome results from too much activity in the serotonin system: this is usually triggered by taking both an SSRI and a second medication that increases serotonin activity, for example, an MAOI. Patients with serotonin syndrome can experience many symptoms including restlessness, agitation, twitching or stiff muscles, a loss of coordination, heavy sweating, shivering, diarrhea, an inability to sleep, and headache. They may have a rapid pulse, high blood pressure, and dilated pupils. If severe they may show a very high temperature, have seizures, or pass out. Severe serotonin syndrome can be fatal.

* Zisook S1, Rush AJ, Haight BR, Clines DC, Rockett CB. Use of bupropion in combination with serotonin reuptake inhibitors. Biol Psychiatry. 2006 Feb 1;59(3):203-10. Epub 2005 Sep 13.

One of the most common causes of serotonin syndrome is a patient taking an antidepressant that increases serotonin such as an SSRI, SNRI, or MAOI, starting treatment with another type of medication that affects serotonin. These can include certain pain killers, anti-migraine drugs, some drugs used for nausea, and even some herbal medicines and over the counter cough medications. Certain illicit drugs including ecstasy, LSD, cocaine and amphetamines can also trigger serotonin syndrome. It is also a common consequence of taking an overdose of an SSRI.

Patients who think they may be developing serotonin syndrome should seek medical help urgently.

A second antidepressant is not the only thing, however, that can be added to an initial antidepressant to try and improve clinical outcomes. There are a number of different types of medications that have been tested as so-called adjuvant therapies. The oldest of these approaches is the use of the medication, lithium. Lithium was initially developed, and is widely used, as a treatment for bipolar disorder. It is a "mood stabilizer" that can help resolve manic or depressive episodes or act to reduce the frequency of the occurrence of either of these extremes. It is typically more commonly effective in the treatment of mania than depression.

The use of lithium in treating depression in patients who do not have bipolar disorder was first investigated in the late 1960's soon after its value in bipolar disorder was discovered. Its application as an adjuvant agent, added to an unsuccessful antidepressant, was first tested in research in the early 1980s with promising outcomes. Since that time, a series of studies, mostly small, have directly tested whether lithium is effective with reasonably consistently positive results. These studies were, however, mainly conducted before the development of SSRIs. Most of the studies show that adding lithium to a TCA antidepressant can help and there are few studies showing that lithium has value when added to more commonly used antidepressants. If lithium helps get you better, it has one other important advantage: it seems to reduce the likelihood of depression recurring to a greater degree than it might when taking an antidepressant alone. This is important given that depression has a nasty habit of coming back. Another advantage of lithium treatment is that it seems to work quickly. If a patient has not responded after 2 weeks of an adequate dose, it is reasonable to stop it and move on to other options.

## Why Doesn't Everyone Just Take Lithium?

If lithium enhances response and keeps patients well for longer, why is it not more widely used? Well, for one, it is an old drug, off patent and relatively cheap, so there is little motivation for pharmaceutical companies to promote its use. Doctors over time have become somewhat de-skilled in its use; they just are not as familiar with how to prescribe and monitor it as doctors were a few decades ago.

It is also not a simple drug to take. Lithium is a basic element (if you can remember your high school science you will recall it is on the periodic table) which is taken in the form of a salt. This means it is processed by the body in very different ways from most other drugs, and has some side effects directly consistent with taking a high dose of salt. Amongst other effects, it will make you thirsty and need to urinate more frequently. It is possible to accurately measure levels of lithium in blood which allows quite precise dosing: we also have a very good idea of how much lithium needs to be in the blood for it to work. This is fortunate as lithium has lots of side effects, especially at higher doses. At doses not far above the effective range, it can also cause serious adverse effects, with damage to the kidneys a major long-term problem for some patients. For these reasons, lithium therapy needs to be carefully monitored and many doctors do not feel confident with what this requires.

Lithium has one additional and profoundly unique advantage: it lowers rates of suicide.* Studies involving tens of thousands of patients with mood problems have consistently shown that it reduces rates of suicide, down to a level close to or equivalent to that seen in the general

* Tom Bschor. Lithium in the Treatment of Major Depressive Disorder. Drugs volume 74, pages855–862(2014)

population. Critically, this effect is seen in both unipolar and bipolar depression: it is just as prominent an effect in depressed patients without bipolar disorder.

The effect is also quite specific to lithium. It is not seen with antidepressants or other mood stabilizers used in the treatment of the bipolar disorder.

### What About Just Adding Lithium to Drinking Water?

Although not directly related to the question of depression treatment, recent research suggests that widespread consumption of higher levels of lithium could have significant benefits across the population in general. Specifically, there is a reduction in rates of dementia in places where higher levels of lithium are naturally found in drinking water!

So, lithium is a very good but a somewhat tricky and underused option. What are the other augmentation choices? Taking doses of thyroid hormone in tablet form is one of these. Thyroid hormone is a substance made in a gland at the front of the neck. As we have already discussed, having too little thyroid hormone can produce significant depressive symptoms. Too much thyroid hormone can look a little like mania. If your body is not making enough thyroid hormone, you definitely need to take this in tablet form to stave off depression along with a variety of serious medical consequences. What if your thyroid levels are actually ok? Well, a number of clinical trials, although again small, have suggested that taking "extra" thyroid hormone in tablet form, can help boost the effects of antidepressant medication and this can mostly be done safely. The overall number of responders to this strategy is probably fairly small and like lithium, it is an approach not promoted widely by pharmaceutical interests.

An approach that has had the well-financed backing of "big pharma" is the use of the so called "atypical" or second-generation antipsychotic drugs. Antipsychotic drugs were first developed in the 1960s for the treatment of schizophrenia. A group of these drugs, relatively similar in effects and often called "typical antipsychotics," were used as the mainstay of the treatment of schizophrenia until the 1990s. During that decade, as the range of antidepressants starting to expand following the development of fluoxetine, a new generation of antipsychotic drugs also began to be released. Over time, many members of this second generation of "atypical" antipsychotics were then evaluated for benefit in other disorders, especially in bipolar disorder and depression, often as the time on their patents for use in schizophrenia started to run down. Drugs such as olanzapine, quetiapine, aripiprazole, and risperidone have been evaluated in trials as adjuvant agents in depression. They seem to offer benefits, but all have fairly serious side effects.

When first marketed for the management of schizophrenia, second generation antipsychotics were heavily promoted as being much safer and better tolerated than the first-generation medications available at the time. The first of these drugs, risperidone, olanzapine and quetiapine, did seem to have fewer side effects when they first came to market. This was due to a combination of factors. First, they were more moderately dosed than the older medications and at the recommended doses produced less muscle stiffness, tremulousness, and abnormal movements. These had been major problems with the older drugs, making them very unpopular with patients.

They also appeared a lot better because the side effects they did cause were much more insidious: instead of producing muscle stiffness and spasms in the first weeks of treatment, some caused weight gain and diabetes, which developed slowly over months. This was not all obvious to the doctors prescribing them, especially early on. They would be started by doctors practicing on the wards of hospital units when patients were admitted with a relapse or flare up of the symptoms of their illness. The issues would become apparent months later, usually to other doctors managing the patient in the community. These doctors would often be between a rock and a hard place: if they took the patients off these medications they risked a relapse and rehospitalization. If not, the side effects accumulated. It took a long time for an understanding of these issues to feedback to the places and psychiatrists where patients were being started on these meds by the thousands.

What were the issues? The biggest one, no pun intended, was weight gain. Patients, especially on olanzapine, could put on 10, 20, or 30kg. They would sometimes wake up at night hungry. Some female patients compared their cravings to being pregnant. With increased weight came an elevated risk of diabetes and all the other health problems associated with increased weight. Other medications increased a hormone called prolactin disrupting sexual function and causing men to develop female looking breasts. Of note, some of the nefarious behaviors of the pharmaceutical industry, best described in a previous chapter regarding Eli Lilly's suppression of information to do with suicidality arising from the use of fluoxetine, reared their ugly head again. And again, the main culprit was Eli Lily. This time it was their failure to be upfront with the data that clearly showed the weight gain and other complications caused by olanzapine.

The use of second-generation antipsychotics as adjuvant agents in depression has been subject of considerable research in studies conducted by the pharmaceutical industry. These studies have shown a consistent benefit of adding an antipsychotic when an antidepressant has not fully worked. Multiple drugs have been supported. However, there are limitations of these studies. The average difference in depression improvement between drug and placebo across trials has been small. A small difference may arise from a sedating drug improving sleep (and hence daytime energy) without really improving the main depressive symptoms. The studies do not show improvement in more general measures such as of the quality of life. The studies have also tended to be short term: they do not address the safety of long-term treatment. These issues have resulted in very different recommendations on use being developed by different professional groups around the world. A reasonable conclusion seems to be that they may have short term benefits, but longer term use should be limited to avoid the accumulating impact of side effects. Certainly, whether a patient benefits from their use or not, the antipsychotic should be weaned and stopped as soon as possible.

So where does this leave us? And where does it leave Anne with whom we started this chapter? Many patients will not respond to initial medication therapy; this is clear. She certainly did not. If this happens, a clear reassessment of the diagnosis is necessary. Is medication the solution to the problem at all? Would the patient be better off with a form of psychotherapy or some other type of medication?

If specific treatment for depression is necessary, there are options. These include switching to another antidepressant, adding a second antidepressant, or one of a number of adjuvant agents. Anne tried the first approach, probably the most common switch, from an SSRI to an SNRI (as well as from one SSRI to another). She also tried an adjuvant antipsychotic. Neither of these approaches worked although these may prove useful for some. Clearly, these options are not foolproof. Back on a SSRI, she had a couple of other options. Switch again, perhaps to an older agent or at least something more substantially different from the SSRIs, start a second antidepressant, lithium, thyroid hormone, or perhaps another antipsychotic. She was not enthused by any of these options. She was actually pretty sick of the idea of more chopping and changing of drugs. So, what else could we do? In the following chapters, we will investigate what the other options are and what they are likely to be in the coming years.

Before we do, I want to briefly touch on one other issue that is increasingly relevant in the choice of medication for patients with depression: that of genetic testing. Anything to do with genetics tends to take on an aura of "hard science," something concrete and certain. Exactly the opposite of how psychiatric treatment is usually perceived. As such, it is tempting to buy into the idea that genetic testing is the solution to what is often a process of trial and error. But how might this work? And is it helpful?

The first approaches to genetic testing and antidepressant treatment took a somewhat indirect approach. Most medications, and certainly most antidepressants, are broken down by specific enzymes in the liver. This process stops medication levels from progressively building up in our bodies over time. The liver breaks down the medications into components which are then most commonly excreted in the urine. The enzymes in the liver, like all proteins in our bodies, are produced from specific genes. These genes can vary, in ways that are fairly well understood, and these variations can affect the function of the enzymes.

There are typically three options: the enzyme can function normally, the enzyme can be over-active, or it can be under-active. In the over or "hyperactive" case, medications metabolized by that enzyme will be broken down faster, meaning the medication will be less active than it would be expected to be at a typical dose (as there will be less of it circulating in the blood). These so called "fast metabolizers" might therefore need a higher dose than usual to get the same helpful medication effect.

The opposite is the case for "slow metabolizers," those with sluggish, under active enzymes. When a patient with this profile takes medication, the levels of this will be higher in their blood. They might, therefore, have a greater rate of side effects. They might repeatedly fail to tolerate prescribed medications, over and over again.

Then there is the possibility that we could understand genes that relate to whether a medication will work; not how much of the medication is in the blood but whether the medication meaningfully interacts in the brain to change something important in depression itself. This is a much bigger challenge as we do not really understand the genes that relate to depression, let alone what might be associated with successful treatment. One shortcut, not requiring a full understanding of the disorder, could be to assess the genetic profiles in many patients who started on medications and just try and find the genes that are more or less expressed in those who get better. It might be possible to find a pattern of genes that are associated with a better response, and can be used to predict this clinically, even if we do not really understand what these genes all do.

This all seems to make a lot of sense. If we can measure the type of genes someone has, we could use this to help choose the medication they take and the dose that is likely to be well tolerated and hopefully effective. Does this really work, however?

The first studies conducted to explore this did show that there seemed to be a pattern of differences in the genetic make-up of medication responders and non-responders. However, this is really not sufficient proof of value. What was required were studies where genetic profiles were assessed and then medication chosen based on the results of these tests. This process could be conducted in one group of patients and the outcomes compared to those seen in patients where genetic testing was not included in the decision making.

A number of these studies have now been conducted. A recent analysis pooled the results of five of these studies.* All five studies tested the effects of multiple genes (between 5 and 30) with all including the major genes involved in medication metabolism/breakdown in the liver. This analysis found that genetic testing was associated with improved outcomes. However, the authors noted that all of these studies were sponsored by companies responsible for the genetic testing and the psychiatrists in these trials were aware of the treatment group that patients were allocated. This opens the door for biases of the psychiatrists to creep in and affect the results.

Where does this leave us? The data suggests these approaches may have value but really require substantial independent testing—studies doing this are now underway. Most importantly, the improvements in outcomes seen in these studies were relatively modest: genetic testing may improve things a bit, but it does not look like it will be the solution to one of the biggest problems: how do we help the many patients for whom medication has not been the answer? This will be our focus in the coming chapters.

* Bousman, C. A., Arandjelovic, K., Mancuso, S. G., Eyre, H. A., & Dunlop, B. W. (2018). Pharmacogenetic tests and depressive symptom remission: a meta-analysis of randomized controlled trials. Pharmacogenomics. doi:10.2217/pgs-2018-0142

# 5

# ECT'S ROLE IN DEPRESSION MANAGEMENT

THERE IS NO more controversial treatment in psychiatry—perhaps in all of medicine—than electroconvulsive therapy, more commonly known as ECT or electric shock treatment. In this chapter, we will explore what ECT is, what are the real advantages of ECT, its problems, and when and how it might have a role in the management of difficult to treat depression.

Before we do, I want to share the story of another patient, whose words and experiences I remember from many years ago as if they were yesterday. This was a patient that I treated while I was a psychiatric trainee, working as a doctor but learning the art and science of psychiatry. In pretty much all medical training, trainees tend to rotate between different jobs to gain experience in varying aspects of the specialty in which they plan to practice. I saw this particular patient very soon after I changed jobs. I had been working in a psychiatric inpatient unit and moved to work on what was referred to as a crisis assessment and treatment team (CAT team). This was a team of doctors, psychiatric nurses, psychologists, and social workers who would treat patients, with usually quite significant mental health problems, in their homes as an alternative to those patients being admitted to hospital.

Soon after I joined the CAT team, I was taken by one of the psychiatric nurses to meet a young female patient who I will call Jane. Jane was 19 years old, about to turn 20. After finishing high school, quite successfully, Jane had taken a gap year to spend backpacking around Europe, a very Australian thing to do. At first, she had a wonderful time. She worked at a pub in London, also fairly typically Australian, and made trips to various European countries. About nine months after arriving in the UK, something profoundly changed. She became markedly withdrawn and was spending most of her time in bed. She had no energy, no motivation to really do anything at all, and had bleak, hopeless thoughts. She had begun to think that life was not worth living, that she would be better off dead, but had not yet formulated a plan or attempted suicide.

Fortunately, Jane had established some good relationships in London, and it was one of her friends who reached out to her parents back in Melbourne to let them know about her plight. Her mother flew to London and arranged for Jane and herself to return to Melbourne within a few days. It was clear to her that something was seriously wrong.

When Jane arrived back, she was taken by her family to her local emergency department who referred her to the CAT team. Thus began the saga of her care. This was about 4 months before I met her. In that time, she was treated with a series of antidepressant medications, brought to her home and supervised by the—as I was to learn, highly dedicated, experienced and well meaning—CAT team doctors and nurses. None of these made any difference at all. When I first met her, she had not left the house for all of those 4 months. She actually had not left her bedroom in all that time, except to go to the bathroom. She had not showered for weeks. Her blinds were closed and had not been opened for ages. She spent all her time in bed, ate small meals in her room, and was not functioning at all.

I was horrified. She is not getting better, "why haven't we been more aggressive with her treatment," I thought and asked, "why is she not in the hospital?" I was determined to change this. My determination, at least for several months, struck up against the stuckness of the situation. Jane and her parents openly accepted her depressive illness and need for treatment. However, they were terrified of her going to the hospital, or trying anything different and just would not agree to this. For another 2 or 3 months, we continued on: medication trials, one after another, with no success. I organized repeated meetings with her parents to try and get them on my side in my desire to be more proactive. This was getting desperate; I saw her fading away. We did not want to act to hospitalize her without her consent, at least her parents support, but for months they did not shift. Eventually, we decided that we had to bite the bullet. She was continuing to lose weight, the situation was just not sustainable and there was no sign of improvement. We told the family that she really had to come into the hospital and would need to try a course of ECT, medication clearly was of no use. They remained reluctant but would not resist and so she was made an involuntary patient, to be treated initially against her wished, and admitted to the hospital.

Two weeks later, I went to the ward to see how she was doing. Following admission, the treatment team had confirmed the diagnosis of depression, and after a few days of assessment, had commenced a course of ECT. She had undergone four treatments by the time I saw her. She had already changed. Almost unrecognizable from the young woman I had seen over and over again in her dark smelly bedroom. She was dressed smartly, made eye contact, smiled, and spoke freely. She described how much better she felt and how she was looking forward to going home. She was not sure if she was having another one or two treatments, but her mood was great.

It was her parting words that have stuck in my mind for over 20 years now. "Why did you wait so long?" In trying to support her wishes, and those of her family, most critically to avoid ECT, we had just prolonged her suffering, far longer than seemed reasonable to her now. ECT had profoundly turned things around for her, in just a matter of days.

This interaction has stayed with me for many years as it was a stark illustration of the potency of ECT and its ability to resolve depression rapidly and with efficacy not seen with any other psychiatric therapies. However, ECT remains controversial: partially for good reasons and partially not. In this chapter I hope to unpack these issues and provide a sensible basis on which you might think about ECT as a treatment for yourself or for someone you care for.

The story of Sylvia Plath is also an extremely informative one that highlights many of the important issues around ECT that we will discuss in the following pages. Plath, in her autobiographical novel *The Bell Jar,* described the horrors of early ECT but also its value when done in a more humane manner. Her death by suicide, during a subsequent episode of depression many years later, also highlights the tragic consequences of the under-treatment of depression.

Plath first had a series of ECT treatments in 1953, done without any of the medications used to effectively and safely support treatment now. She described this experience in vivid terms:

*"Then something bent down and took hold of me and shook me like the end of the world. Whee-ee-ee-ee-ee, it shrilled, through an air crackling with blue light, and with each flash a great jolt drubbed me till I thought my bones would break and the sap fly out of me like a split plant. I wondered what terrible thing it was that I had done."\**

*Her subsequent experience with "modified ECT" was much different. She awakes from her first treatment and describes "All the heat and fear purged itself. I felt surprisingly at peace."* She continued this treatment course until fully recovered and was well for many years afterward. When Plath experienced a relapse of depression a decade later, she only received medication treatment and ultimately ended her own life, something it has been argued could have been prevented by a further course of ECT.\*\*

So how did we get to a place where we have this extremely effective treatment with such a bad rep? Well to understand this requires at least a little historical detour and an appreciation of differences in the treatments experienced by Plath.

The idea of inducing seizures to treat mental illness was first proposed by Ladislas Meduna in Budapest in the 1920s, following an observation that patients who experienced seizures had a temporary reduction in the severity of psychotic symptoms, the hallucinations and delusions experienced by patients with schizophrenia. Meduna experimented with drug-induced seizures, initially by injections of camphor oil and then via the oral administration of pentylenetetrazol (Metrazol). The latter

* Sylvia Plath, 1981, pp. 117–118; *The Bell Jar* by Sylvia Plath. Copyright © 1971 by Harper & Row, Publishers, Inc.
** Sylvia Plath Recovered Completely by Electroconvulsive Therapy at the Age of 21 Years and Might Have Been Saved by Another Series 9 Years Later Bergsholm, Per MD, PhD The Journal of ECT: September 2017 - Volume 33 - Issue 3 - p e26

drug produced seizures rapidly but also a terrible sense of dread that was feared greatly by patients.

ECT was developed as a hopefully more humane method of seizure induction, by Ugo Cerletti and Lucio Bini in Rome in the 1930s. After testing electrical seizure induction in dogs, they commenced testing in patients with schizophrenia, the group that had been the focus of Meduna's work as well. The use of ECT was first prescribed publicly in 1938 and its use spread rapidly in Europe and to North America by the mid 1940's.

Although the extent and rapidity of the spread of ECT suggests that there must have been some evidence of effectiveness driving its uptake, it is important to be aware of the context of its introduction. By the 1930s, asylums around the world were overflowing with patients who were often housed in terrible conditions and who suffered disorders for which there were no effective treatments. The use of insulin coma therapy and leucotomy (surgical lobotomy usually performed without anesthesia) also spread rapidly at the same time without decent evidence of effectiveness outweighing marked risks. One notable trend in the early years of the use of ECT was the extension of its use into the treatment of other mental health conditions, especially depression. This rapidly became a common reason for its application internationally.

The way ECT was first used, in "unmodified form," had major problems. Seizures were induced in awake patients which was extremely painful and distressing, and the electrical stimulus and seizures could produce fractures in the limbs and spine. It was this form of ECT that was portrayed in the film "One flew over the Cuckoo's nest." This was released in 1975 but portrayed ECT from the 1950's.* It also highlighted that ECT was at times used in a punitive manner and it helped develop a perception of ECT that has profoundly shaped the way that the public sees ECT up until the modern day. This has not been helped by the continued resurrection of the movie as a way of portraying the treatment. For example, an article in a Canadian newspaper in 2013

---

* The movie was based on the book by Ken Kesey which was released in 1962. Kesey had worked in a mental hospital in the 1950s.

presented an image from the movie as a modern representation of ECT, not in its correct historical context.

The form of ECT used in the 1950s has as little in common with modern day ECT as a World War II battlefield amputation would have with a modern surgical procedure. Presentation of the treatment in this misleading manner does a great disservice to patients like Jane and her family who have to weigh up whether this is the right treatment for them.

Through the 1960s and 1970s the use of ECT increased dramatically, as psychotropic medications became widely available and became the mainstay of medical psychiatric treatment. However, during this time the procedure was gradually refined and substantially improved. The first step was the introduction of medication to induce muscle paralysis, to lessen the risk of fractures. Drugs were then introduced to relax the patient pre-treatment, and later the use of full anesthesia. The treatment was slowly transforming into something more closely resembling a modern medical procedure. These changes, however, were not really reflected in the way ECT was viewed in the broader community, its use was especially criticized by the anti-psychiatry movement and later in campaigns by certain religious groups.

Beyond the introduction of anesthesia and muscle relaxation, ECT methods have continued to be refined over the last couple of decades. One of these advances is especially worthy of note and has placed the modern use of ECT on a much firmer scientific footing. I am referring here to a series of randomized controlled trials that have introduced and tested a series of methods to maximize effectiveness while trying to limit the most troublesome of ECT side effects, memory impairment. There have been several related advances tested in these trials: improving the nature of the electrical current used, personalizing the dose of electricity used, and developing new electrode placements.

In regard to the former, the electrical current used for ECT has changed over time from a "sine wave," where the current varies over time relatively gradually, to a so called "square wave" pulse sequence. During the application of a square wave pulse, the full strength of the current comes on much more rapidly, which proves a more efficient way of inducing seizures. More efficient means lower doses are needed and hence fewer side effects. More recent decades have seen the testing of "brief pulse" and then "ultra-brief pulse" ECT. These involve the use of shorter pulses of electricity, pulses that again more efficiently induce a seizure and with a less overall "dose" of electricity applied to the brain.

Alongside these developments has been a realization that the strength of the electrical current, the "dose", required to produce optimal benefits, is not the same for all patients and should be tailored to the type of ECT being delivered. This has led to the widespread introduction of a process to assess the optimal dose at the outset of a course of ECT for each patient. To do this, during the first ECT session, electrical stimuli are applied at a gradually increasing dose, until a seizure is produced. The minimum dose required to produce a seizure is an individual patient's "seizure threshold." The electrical current used for the course of treatment is then a multiple of this threshold: for example, 1½ times, 3 times, or 6 times seizure threshold. In this way, the optimal dose is determined for each patient and specifically for the type of ECT being used.

As well as altering the pulse current and the dose, researchers were busy refining electrode placement. ECT was initially done by placing the two electrodes on either side of the head, over the position of the temporal lobes of the brain: *bitemporal ECT*. Importantly, one part of the brain that sits inside the temporal lobe is an unusually shaped area called the hippocampus. The hippocampus is a critical structure for memory, and it was clear early in the use of ECT that bitemporal ECT could cause marked memory impairment. Two significant improvements in bitemporal ECT are in use today. These are *right unilateral ECT* and *bifrontal ECT*. In the former, the two electrodes are both placed on the right side of the head: this reduces somewhat the degree of hippocampal stimulation, especially when combined with the use of ultra-brief pulses. Bifrontal ECT involves the placement of the two electrodes across the frontal area of the brain, again further away from the temporal lobes.

A series of studies have compared these forms of ECT and led to a progressive refinement of practice. Ultra-brief right unilateral ECT (at six times the seizure threshold) seems to have the best side effect profile, followed by bifrontal and brief pulse right unilateral ECT with bitemporal ECT having the worst effects on memory. The order is somewhat reversed in regard to efficacy although the unilateral forms of ECT have efficacy not much worse than bitemporal ECT if the right dosing approach is used.

What is typically used in clinical practice tends to vary somewhat by treating psychiatrist, patient characteristics, and the location of care. Ultra-brief right unilateral ECT has become a very common first-line treatment for most patients, although there are still some concerns that a course of this may take a little longer than a course of other forms of ECT. Bitemporal ECT is still used, although much less commonly: usually in situations where an extremely urgent clinical response is required, for example in a patient who has stopped eating and drinking or is highly suicidal.

Despite these improvements, there are still significant side effect problems with ECT. Using anesthesia is an essential advance to maximize the safety of ECT but there is always some risk with a general anesthetic, including very rarely the death of the patient. Patients can experience a variety of other problems such as headaches and muscle aches and pains. The most critical issue, however, remains that of memory impairment.

## Types of Memory

Psychologists and cognitive neuroscientists describe different forms of memory and memory impairment, sometimes with a confusing range of terms. For our purposes in this chapter we will talk about the following:

- **Short-term memory:** The ability to remember things over relatively limited periods of time: seconds to minutes.
- **Long-term memory:** The ability to recall things from one's past, a timescale of minutes to years.
- **Retrograde amnesia:** An inability to remember things that happened before the onset of memory problems.
- **Anterograde amnesia:** An ongoing inability to remember things/problems with laying down new memories.

ECT can be responsible for several types of memory impairment, and these are worth considering separately. By far the most common pattern of memory impairment seen in a patient having ECT is trouble remembering the events of the day when the patient has had an ECT treatment, especially the hours immediately following treatment. A more severe pattern is seen where this extends for the full day of treatment, or even across the weeks that the patient is having ECT. Memory for these times will not come back: the experience of these hours, days or weeks are lost.

Some patients say that this is not really that much of a problem. They are having trouble remembering a time they are quite happy to forget. Hours or days when they were miserable, hospitalized, not themselves. However, this is far from a universal experience. Some people will find any sense of disruption of their memory, their personal narrative, really distressing. Others are just understandably upset about their inability to remember important things that might happen during this time, such as a birthday or important appointment. They might question "what did I do?" "Did I say something embarrassing to someone?"

Patients are almost universally more concerned if this inability to remember new things (anterograde amnesia) extends beyond the end of the ECT treatment: if days, weeks, months or years post ECT they find themselves still struggling to remember new things. Certainly, ECT seems to cause this in the short term. It is less clear whether more persistent problems are attributable to ECT. The research on this is hard to interpret. Patients who continue to experience depression post ECT will likely have some degree of memory impairment arising from their depression which confuses the research studies. Personally, this is not something I have seen much of in the many patients I have seen who have had courses of ECT in the past. It does not lessen, however, the experiences of patients who describe this effect and the anguish it may cause them.

The form of memory impairment that is perhaps feared most by patients is a disruption of long-term memory: a situation where patients cannot recall important elements of their past: perhaps their childhood memories or the names of people they have known. Whether this is actually caused by ECT has been a controversial notion for many years.

It was doubted and at times denied by psychiatry. The situation was not really helped by the challenges of doing research in this area. It can be difficult to reliably test long-term memory: the assessor really does not have any magic way of looking into the person's past to interrogate what they should have remembered.

In my view, it is quite clear. ECT can cause this sort of long-term memory disruption, although it does not do so commonly. I have seen too many patients who have had dramatic changes in their capacity to recall important elements of their past life to think that this is not the case. These patients are, fortunately, only a small subset of the patients who have ECT and I think this problem is relatively rare: certainly, much rarer than the issues experienced remembering things around the time of treatment. In my experience, these problems have also been most common in certain patients: young patients and those having multiple courses of ECT or long-term ongoing maintenance ECT.

There are some other elements that might provide some predictive guidance on whether ECT related memory impairment is likely to be a problem. Most commonly, there appears to be a relationship between what is called disorientation immediately after treatment and the likelihood of memory issues. Most patients will wake up from a general anesthetic slightly confused, a little unclear about where they are and what has happened. After an ECT treatment, this is usually worse. At times, the confusion, "I don't know where I am, what day it is, what has happened," extends out in time. The longer this time, the more likely the patient will experience the other sorts of memory issues we have discussed. If a patient is experiencing prolonged periods of disorientation after the first few ECT treatments, this might be a reason for stopping ECT or trying a more memory sparing type if there is another sensible treatment option to choose.

As I indicated above, maintenance ECT is often more commonly associated with memory problems. Maintenance ECT refers to the ongoing use of ECT, usually at less frequent intervals, to prevent depression from returning. ECT is usually provided three times per week when initially treating depression. After a patient responds, they will often have a short period of treatment where the therapy is weaned or titrated down: for example, two sessions per week for one or two weeks and then maybe one session a week for a short time. This may then be extended into maintenance. The frequency of sessions will be gradually reduced, if possible, to one every two to four weeks. There is not a great deal of high quality research evidence that maintenance ECT is effective. However, it is commonly used as sometimes patients just do not have any other options: their depression returns quickly even with medication and psychotherapy when ECT is stopped.

I would like to share a striking example of the dilemma this can create. "Rachel" was a 38-year-old mother of two when we first met. She had first experienced depression at age 19 which eventually responded to antidepressant medication, the third one she tried. She stayed on the medication for about a year and did well after stopping. In her 20s she completed two university degrees and had two children, a boy and girl. Her troubles began after the birth of her second child. She developed an intense relapse of depression, initially diagnosed as post-partum depression. Over the next 2½ years she underwent extensive medication therapy. This included the medication that had worked for her the first time, several SSRIs, two SNRIs, a tricyclic antidepressant, three other antidepressants, lithium, and several antipsychotics. Nothing made any difference at all. Not a bit. She engaged with an experienced psychologist and undertook cognitive behavioral therapy to no avail. She had three admissions to the hospital during this time, two in response to suicidal ideation.

On the third admission, a decision was taken to try ECT, and she had a course of right unilateral ECT. She responded very well to nine treatments but relapsed soon after discharge. This led to readmission, a further ten ECT, and a second recovery. After this admission, fearful of another relapse, Rachel agreed to commence maintenance ECT which she subsequently did. This began weekly, then once every two weeks. After a few months, her psychiatrist tried to reduce further, but by the third week without treatment, Rachel's symptoms were starting to creep back. Treatment increased in frequency again until it seemed reasonable to try and space it out once more: every time this was tried, however, the same result ensued. It looked like Rachel was stuck with treatment every two weeks.

Treatment this regularly did seem to control her depression. However, at a considerable cost. During her initial two courses of treatment, Rachel had suffered memory problems but there was always a sense that these would be temporary. She was willing to put up with this to get better. However, now that she was having treatment continually, the memory effects, if anything, seemed to add up over time. She was now pretty much experiencing a continual incapacity to remember any new information. She could remember her past without a problem, however, it was as if everything stopped when she started the ECT. She could not remember anything meaningful after that time. This went on for over five years. Multiple attempts were made to reduce the ECT, to change the type of ECT, but nothing worked. She was stuck. Her choice was to either be profoundly depressed or live in a twilight world where one day was not linked to the next.

She described the most profound effect of this many years later when she had stopped ECT and fortunately found a way to achieve a period of prolonged wellness. She had recovered her capacity to remember new things but the years of ECT were a complete blank. During the time of her ECT, she had moved with her family to another city and lived there for two years, subsequently returning to her hometown. When she was well again her husband took her back to where she had lived for those two years, to the family home, and to the school her children had gone to. She could recall none of it: it was like she was seeing it all for the first time.

There is one more problem with ECT that is worthy of further discussion. As alluded to already, ECT is just about the most stigmatized therapy in all of medicine. Patients without direct experience of ECT will almost universally have quite negative views about ECT. I have lost count of the times "one flew over the cuckoo's nest" has come up in discussions about the treatment. This one book and movie are not solely to blame: there are many negative, and very few balanced portrayals of ECT, in any form of media. However, it is unlikely that there is one representation of any medical treatment that has so profoundly affected the views of people about that treatment, certainly not for so many years. The carers of patients will share these negative views, as will many doctors, both within and outside of psychiatry. Fortunately, there have been some balanced descriptions of ECT that prospective patients can access and read, although these are generally drowned out in any typical Google search. Kitty Dukakis, the wife of former US presidential candidate Michael Dukakis, wrote a detailed description of her battle with depression and addiction and the curative power of ECT in a book in 2007 with journalist Larry Tye.* In this she was able to reflect on both the benefits and challenges of ECT:

*"That isn't to say that ECT is either a panacea or without flaws—but when used in the right way for the right purposes it's of great benefit, and condemning it because it isn't perfect would lead to more suffering and harm, no less."*

The descriptions of her experiences, and Rachel's story, provide valuable lessons on some of the benefits and challenges of ECT. It was the only thing that helped Rachel to get well and stay well, but this came at a cost, almost as disabling as her depression. Fortunately, many patients—like Jane, who we met earlier—do a lot better with ECT, and many respond without substantial side effects. It has been vilified and attacked repeatedly for many years. However, it will be the patients who ultimately suffer if ECT is made less available, not the religious zealots calling for its abolition. There are considerable, and quite reasonable, concerns about the use of ECT in patients who are unable to consent (see below). However, in patients who are providing fully informed consent, ECT remains a valuable, if still a problematic therapy. Clearly though, it will not be the solution for many patients: we need many more effective options. In the coming chapters we will explore what some of these are.

---

* Shock: The Healing Power of Electroconvulsive . . . (Paperback)by Kitty Dukakis, Larry Tye, Avery, New York, 2007

## Involuntary ECT

If the use of ECT is controversial, its use in patients who have not provided informed consent generates even more concern. The use of involuntary ECT conjures up images of mind control and of medically sanctioned punishment. It also raises legitimate concerns about how the provision of a treatment with serious side effects, which can be highly personally impactful, can be ethically justified in the absence of consent. However, at times psychiatrists have to address the management of very ill patients with depression. These patients can experience persistent and intrusive suicidal ideation and at times patients may even stop eating and drinking. They might become mute, not able to respond and engage in a nuanced discussion of therapeutic options. Many patients who have reached this level of severity will struggle to be able to provide true consent. Under these circumstances, ECT may be the only viable lifesaving treatment. Withholding therapy due to concerns about consent may prove fatal.

# 6

# TRANSCRANIAL MAGNETIC STIMULATION IN THE MODERN MANAGEMENT OF DEPRESSION

EILEEN WAS APPROACHING her 67th birthday when her psychiatrist called me on the phone. He had been treating her for many years and was really stuck. Could we help? For years she had been battling depression and all attempts at treatment had proved futile. However, there was one thing that had yet to be tried, transcranial magnetic stimulation (TMS).

Eileen first struggled with depression back in her early 20s. She had an episode that persisted for about 18 months, at that time and then another in her late 30s. She recovered from both of these and in between, led an enjoyable and active life. She worked for a long period of time as a seamstress and had a family of three children: two boys and a girl. After the episode in her late 30s, she remained well for another 10 years, living life free of any concerns about depression. However, as her menopause began, a common risk time for women with a history of depression, she experienced a prolonged and nasty relapse. She felt overwhelmed by life most of the time and hopeless about the future. She required hospitalization for the first time as she struggled with waves of suicidal thoughts. She did not want to die and devastate her family but would get intrusive and persistent thoughts of crashing her car on the freeway. She spent about a month in the hospital and eventually was able to leave on antidepressant medication, but only really recovered in part.

Over the next 15 years, she seemed to struggle more often than not. She had multiple episodes of depression that seemed to take longer to get better each time, and which became increasingly more frequent. In between episodes, she would not quite fully get back the joy of life that she once had known. Was this the depression lingering, the impact of her recurrent episodes on her confidence and self-esteem, or a side effect of the medication? It wasn't clear. She was on a merry-go-round of antidepressant medications, all the usual suspects. Prozac, Effexor, Cymbalta, Avanza, Zoloft, Citalopram. Her psychiatrist tried adding Lithium, Abilify, Zyprexa, Seroquel, and Lamictal. There were better periods, sometimes for up to six or nine months, but some pretty lousy times as well. The worst episodes would eventually resolve but she was left with a sense of dread, just waiting for the black cloud to return. Eventually, it did, and then her medication was changed again, and again, and again.

Not long after she turned sixty, she had ECT for the first time. Medication was not working during an especially long and troublesome period of depression and her family and doctor were very worried about her. After the usual medication change did not work, she underwent nine unilateral right-sided ECT. This, fortunately, was successful. Her depression quickly abated. She also tolerated the ECT reasonably well: she had some mild memory problems for a week or two but that was all.

She went home and tried to get on with life. Her relief, however, was short lived. Depression returned fairly quickly and within 10 weeks she was back in the hospital. She recommenced ECT and responded again, in pretty much the same way. This time, maintenance ECT was proposed. It was suggested that she come back to the hospital as a day patient, initially once per week and then with gradually reducing frequency. She started the maintenance with her fingers crossed. Ongoing ECT certainly helped to some degree. Her mood remained more stable than before, with no major relapse over the following six months. She was not out of the woods yet, however. The memory problems which had been tolerable during the short-term periods of treatment were much more problematic now. Her experience of this was similar to that of Rachel's, who we met in Chapter 5. With the persistent ECT, she felt clouded a lot of the time. It was always worse for a few days after each treatment but never quite felt like it completely went away. She really hated this. She also had a couple of falls. She saw her GP who sent her to a neurologist. He had her undergo an electroencephalogram (EEG). An EEG involves placing a series of recording electrodes across the scalp to measure brain waves, just as an electrocardiogram (ECG) is used to measure the waves of electricity from the heart. The EEG was not completely normal: there were abnormal patterns of electrical activity. It was not definitive, and a follow-up brain scan was normal but the neurologist suggested that these changes might be coming from the ECT and that it should be stopped.

Predictably, over the next 2 months, her mood deteriorated, and she was soon back in the hospital. She tried another couple of medications and was then referred to us, still very depressed. When I saw her for the first time, she was feeling really very hopeless. She felt that she was going to be depressed forever and suicidal thoughts were a constant presence. She did not want to hurt her family, especially her three daughters, and was worried about the impact killing herself would have on her children and grandchildren but felt like it was just too hard to keep living. She had trouble spending time out of bed during the day, and had no interest in her hobbies or really anything else. Although she spent most of her time in bed, she had trouble sleeping. When she did, she woke unrefreshed, like it was the end of a long day. She did not feel like eating and felt weighed down, flat and lethargic.

Eileen came to see me with really no sense of hope that anything was going to help, and the referral from her psychiatrist also gave the impression that he did not hold out much hope of anything making a substantial difference. I had something to offer but did not want to create a false sense of expectation in Eileen or her family. This thing, TMS, certainly could work as an antidepressant. By the time I saw Eileen, I was convinced of that, but could it help someone struggling as much as she was?

TMS is unlike anything else used in the treatment of depression. It involves a form of stimulation of the brain, like ECT, but it does not produce a seizure. Unlike ECT, TMS does not involve stimulation with an electrical current: in contrast, it involves the use of a powerful magnetic field. Patients undergoing the procedure sit in a reclining chair whilst the machine "taps away" on their head, providing thousands of magnetic stimuli every day, usually over 15 to 30 minutes. This is nothing like the magnetic wristbands some people wear or put under their pillows. A TMS machine actually takes an electrical current, builds this up to a substantial level in a bank of capacitors, and releases the current, very rapidly, through a coil of electrical wires placed over the scalp. The electrical wires do not come into contact with the body so there is no direct electrical stimulation of the brain.

As it turns out, by some quirk of physics, a changing electrical current like this produces a strong magnetic field. The physics behind this was first described by the English scientist Michael Faraday in 1831: hence, Faraday's law of induction. The magnetic field can pass across the skin and skull into the brain. Just as the changing electrical current in the coil produces a magnetic field, the opposite is also true: a changing magnetic field can induce an electrical current in something that conducts electricity. Our brains happen to be full of things that do this. Our neurons or nerve cells. Therefore, a strong enough magnetic field produced by a strong enough electrical current will produce a flow of electricity in the brain. The outcome of this is to make a group of nerve cells fire.

This effect is actually readily demonstrable. This is done by activating the coil at a high enough level over the "motor cortex," the area of the brain that controls our muscles. When you do this, for example, by stimulating the area of the brain controlling muscles in one of your hands, the nerves controlling the muscles underneath the coil are activated in the brain under the coil. The firing of these nerve cells produces a signal that travels down the spinal cord and arm until a twitch is produced in the hand, all in a matter of a few milliseconds. Depending on how high the machine is turned up, this might be a gentle twitch, barely felt by the person, or a response that is much stronger. At high levels, the whole hand or even arm can seemingly jump out of the control of the person whose brain is being stimulated.

I can still remember the first time it happened to me. The stimulation of the coil produces a sensation on your head, like someone tapping you with a pen or flicking the scalp with an elastic band. At almost the same time, there is a noticeable twitch in the hand on the opposite side of your body, it is moved involuntarily, as if by magic.

The principles underlying TMS were first described over 100 years ago. It took, however, until the 1980s before it was possible to build a machine that could generate a magnetic field that was strong enough, and focused enough, to activate nerve cells through the scalp. These machines were not built with any intent to treat disorders like depression. The first machines, built in Sheffield in the UK, were developed as a way to explore nerve function, by activating the "muscle areas" of the brain and measuring the twitches produced. Scientists could use this technique to study nerve pathways from the brain to other parts of the body. This application of TMS developed rapidly and thousands of research studies have been conducted over the last forty years using these techniques to help understand the normal function of the brain and how it goes awry in various illness states.

Relatively soon after TMS was invented, it was noted that if TMS pulses were applied repeatedly, they could change brain activity. If pulses were repeated very quickly, one after another, usually between five to twenty times per second, they would transiently increase the activity of the area of the brain stimulated. If the researchers went too far, they would sometimes cause a subject to have a seizure, like someone with epilepsy does, as this increase in activity would lead to nerve cells starting to fire by themselves. This slowed down the research that was being done until adequate safety guidelines were established, but these soon were and the amount of research utilizing TMS escalated dramatically over the following years.

As well as increasing brain activity, researchers also found that they could do the opposite. If the pulses were applied much more slowly, usually about one pulse per second, the effect was to reduce, rather than increase brain activity. Using these two approaches, called high and low frequency stimulation, we now had tools that could be used to selectively tune up and tune down areas of the brain and the corresponding brain functions, something barely dreamt of before.

As you would expect, it did not take long before people started to explore the potential beneficial effects of TMS as a therapy for a range of disorders originating from the brain. Depression was the first cab off the rank. This was partially historical: there was an established practice of using ECT in treating depression, so doctors were used to thinking about its treatment from a brain stimulation perspective. It was also a matter of timing. At the time when TMS was becoming available, so was the possibility of using new tools to study brain activity. In particular, positron emission tomography (PET) scanners were starting to be used to help uncover some of the hidden secrets of the brain.

Doing a PET scan involves injecting a radiotracer, a slightly radioactive material which has been attached to something that goes to a place in the body that you want to study. In this case, glucose or sugar is used. Cells in the brain that are active and firing take up glucose as their source of energy. The radiotracer is carried to these cells along with the glucose and the signal from the radiotracer can be detected showing where this has happened. When PET scan studies are done of the brain and its functions, researchers can map areas of the brain that are under or overactive, as they take up more or less glucose than other areas of the brain.

The first studies that were done with PET imaging in patients with depression revealed one fairly consistent finding: that the left prefrontal cortex, a moderate sized area at the front of the brain on the left side, was relatively consistently underactive in patients with depression. This area of the brain is involved in a number of aspects of thinking, including our ability to hold information in mind, and to plan and think sequentially. It is also thought to be involved in complex networks with deeper brain structures that are probably more directly involved in emotional experiences such as sadness.

It is possible that dysfunction of activity in this area of the brain is primarily responsible for depression: that it is failing to control deeper emotional brain regions in people who are depressed leading to over-activity of these "emotional" areas and the experience of depression. The opposite might also be true: that over-activity in emotional brain areas might result in signals shutting down the frontal brain regions. A third possibility is that these areas of the brain are structurally or functionally disconnected. That the problem is related to the connections between brain regions.

Based on these early imaging studies, it was proposed that high frequency or "activating" TMS could be applied to this left frontal region in the treatment of patients with depression. This is one of the few times in the field of psychiatry where a treatment has been developed with a specific hypothesis based on research evidence. This has certainly not been the case with most types of medications used in psychiatry, the precursors of which have mostly been discovered by chance.

Several research groups set out to test this idea. Separate groups, at Harvard University and the National Institutes for Mental Health in Washington DC, conducted two small clinical trials in the mid-1990s. Both studies suggested that TMS might have beneficial effects on depressed patients. From here, research groups in many countries set out to conduct placebo controlled studies, comparing "true" TMS to a fake or placebo treatment, often called sham stimulation.

Although not all of these studies showed benefits (the initial studies were often small and small studies are notoriously unreliable), most did and gradually the beneficial effects were recognized. However, it took another 10 years, until the mid-2000s, for the type of large study to be conducted that would ultimately lead to the approval of the technique by regulatory authorities. This was conducted by a company called Neuronetics Ltd. and the results of this trial were used in a successful application for device approval to the US regulatory agency, the FDA. By 2008 the Neuronetics TMS device was on the market in the US and the era of clinical use of TMS had begun in earnest. At the time of writing, five other TMS devices have been approved in the US and device approvals for various TMS machines have also been granted in countries around the world.

By the time Eileen presented for treatment, I had been running a clinical and research TMS program for almost ten years. Over this time, we conducted a number of clinical trials. These were initially focused on helping to prove that TMS was an effective treatment, but then the focus of our research shifted to exploring alternative ways to apply the treatment that could enhance its effectiveness. Some of this research was ongoing and Eileen agreed to take part in one of these clinical studies. The study was comparing response rates between two different forms of TMS. One was the standard type of activating TMS applied to the front left side of the brain. The other approach was quite different. It involved applying "'low frequency" TMS, the type that reduces brain activity, to the opposite side of the brain, also at the front.

This alternative approach was supported by a different type of brain imaging from the PET scan studies I discussed above. Somewhat after the use of PET became common, it was discovered that Magnetic Resonance Imaging (MRI) machines could be used to take pictures of the functioning of the brain. As well as taking highly detailed pictures of the structure of the brain, they could also be used to detect changes in the oxygen levels in the blood. Oxygen levels change as brain areas are activated as active brain cells need to take up more oxygen than ones at rest.

These functional MRI studies—conducted by us and others—showed that patients with depression seemed to have overactivity in the right side of the brain. This overactivity was seen when the patients were compared to healthy individuals, not at rest, but when performing some thinking tasks. This was in contrast to the underactivity seen on the left in the resting PET scans. Therefore, it made sense to think about applying the "deactivating" low frequency form of TMS to this right side of the brain, and this was what Eileen happened to receive.

As it turned out, I had been quite committed to research developing this right sided TMS approach since I first started to study TMS in depression. This was for a number of quite diverse reasons. First, the idea of targeting right sided changes in the brain appealed to me as I suspected that the studies showing changes on the right during brain activity might be more reflective of what is really going awry in the brains of patients with depression than what the studies at rest were showing. I did not think scans at rest truly compared brain activity between depressed individuals and healthy controls as depressed patients would not be "resting" in the same way (but perhaps thinking negative depressive thoughts).

The other reasons were more down to earth. Left sided treatment at high frequency was more uncomfortable for some patients than low frequency, right sided treatment. Left sided could feel more like a mini jackhammer compared to a gentle tapping. Patients would often describe it as being like having a woodpecker trying to drill a hole into your head. Left sided high frequency TMS was also more likely to induce a seizure than low frequency right sided treatment as it was making the brain more, rather than less, active. Although we know now that this is extremely rare, in the early 2000s it was still something that we were very concerned about.

Then there were issues with the equipment itself. Running high frequency stimulation placed considerably greater stress on the early TMS machines which we were pushing pretty hard, treating multiple patients each day. We seemed to get more breakdowns with high frequency stimulation—there were these capacitor boxes that would suddenly spark, smell very bad, and stop working. The fact that they then needed to be shipped to the other side of the world to be repaired was not insignificant. Then there were the flashing lights with each pulse: in the room, in the corridor, and most problematically, in the hospital meeting room next door! The early machines needed to draw so much electricity to produce the TMS pulses that it literally affected circuits in a decent area of the building. I was not popular when an important meeting coincided with TMS!

Last but not least, the coils we used heated up to a point where they would stop working and had to be cooled down. This happened much quicker with the left sided treatment. With this, we would need to swap the coil two or three times during each treatment. We would have three coils: one on the patient and two hanging in front of an air-conditioning unit running at full speed. The room was very cold, the patient colder (but at least under a blanket) and I was the coldest, standing holding the coil (yes this was before fancy coil stands) right in the cold air blast!

Things were not quite as primitive by the time Eileen presented for her treatment. I was no longer holding the coil and we had a nurse providing the treatment which was administered through a coil held in a stand that was kept cool through an internal fluid system, so at least the room was comfortable. The TMS procedure she underwent began with a measurement of her "resting motor threshold," a procedure conducted to establish how high the machine would be turned up for her treatment. To do this, TMS pulses were applied to the muscle area of her brain until we could work out the lowest pulse strength that would produce a twitch in a muscle in one of her hands.

This measurement is used to work out how high to turn the machine up and also to provide a way to work out where the coil should be placed for treatment. The procedure we were using at the time when Eileen had TMS to determine the coil placement is regarded as a little bit out of date now. When researchers first dreamt up doing TMS for depression, they had to work out a way to find the prefrontal cortex, the area identified in brain scans as being abnormal in patients. They already knew how to find the muscle area: by moving the coil around over the surface of the head and trying to find the spot that produces a muscle twitch. When they looked at brain scans, they saw that the prefrontal cortex was about 5cm in front of the motor area. Therefore, they reasoned, you could simply measure 5cm across the top of the head to work out where to put the coil for treatment.

If this sounds quite simplistic, it is. It is also quite likely to result in incorrect coil placement in many people as head size varies quite considerably between people. More modern approaches to this measurement are based on head size or even brain scans and sophisticated equipment to establish accurately where the coil should be placed. These approaches seem to produce better responses and are increasingly being used widely in clinical practice.

After Eileen's motor threshold was measured and her treatment site worked out, the treatment was prescribed, and she was handed over to a TMS nurse to undergo her first treatment. To have the treatment, she sat in a comfortable reclining chair with her head resting on a pillow to try to keep it still. The coil, which looks a bit like a large old-fashioned key head, but much bigger, was placed over the front of her head and held in place by a stand. The machine was then turned on. The low frequency TMS that Eileen was receiving involved stimulation with one pulse per second for 20 minutes. Just like a clock ticking, she would feel a tapping on her forehead. She could also feel a twitch down the front of her face, above and around her eye. This was about all, however. Low frequency TMS is usually extremely well-tolerated, and some patients even fall asleep during the treatment. High frequency TMS, in contrast, produces a stronger sensation as a large number of pulses are applied in a very short period of time: usually 40 or 50 in four to five seconds. This can give a much stronger sensation. Underneath the coil, the pulsing can even be somewhat painful.

If someone needs to be treated at a high intensity, the nursing staff will usually start at lower levels to allow the patient to get used to the sensation before it is progressively increased. If this is done carefully, most patients will be able to undergo a course of treatment and tolerate TMS extremely well. Fortunately, treatment dropouts are quite rare and certainly less common than with antidepressant medication treatment or ECT.

Eileen would now come to the TMS treatment room to have therapy on a daily basis, five days per week. All patients are told not to expect a great deal initially. Most patients do not notice any change in the first one to two weeks, and the response can take even longer. Eileen's response was fortunately positive and actually fairly stereotypical. Towards the end of the second week of treatment, she noticed a gradual brightening in her mood. She felt more able to concentrate on things and started reading a bit more and doing handicrafts. Over the next week, her mood progressively lifted. By the time she finished her 17th treatment, she was feeling remarkably better, pretty much back to her old self. She was anxious to get out of the hospital and get on with life. We finished up the last couple of treatments, of a planned course of 20, and she went home.

Pleasingly, this type of response to TMS is seen in a decent number of patients. Clinical trials suggest that the response rate to TMS is at least 40 and 50 percent: 4 or 5 patients out of every 10 who have treatment, and may well be higher. The TMS programs that I have been involved in running over the last two decades have treated several thousand patients and through these programs, we have consistently seen an excellent response to TMS in at least half of the patients we treat. In addition to this, a smaller group of patients get a much more limited benefit and about one in three patients do not respond at all. We consider this a considerable success, especially given the fact that, like Eileen, many, if not most of our patients, have had long histories of depression and tried many previous treatments.

At the time of Eileen's treatment, providing TMS to patients who had not responded well to ECT was actually quite uncommon. For many years, I regarded patients not responding to ECT as unlikely to get better with TMS. Eileen didn't fall strictly into this category, but in recent years, we have treated quite a few patients who have received a minimal benefit with ECT and initially somewhat surprisingly to me, quite a few of these have responded well to TMS. I still think that overall ECT is a more effective treatment—the percentage of patients who will respond to ECT is probably higher than the percentage overall who respond to TMS. However, TMS and ECT are quite different approaches and should both be considered in patients with depression struggling to get better. It is also quite likely that the effectiveness of TMS will improve over time as we improve the technique, for example with better targeting and also the possibility of developing a more personalized treatment approaches, adapted treatment in multiple ways specifically for each patient. Lots of research is currently going on to improve the application of TMS in these ways.

There has been considerable debate in the TMS community as to whether patients like Eileen, who have failed many medication treatments, are suitable for TMS or whether it is a more useful treatment approach in patients who are much earlier in the course of their illness, perhaps after they have only failed one or two antidepressants. Some clinical trial data suggest that there might be a slightly better response rate in patients earlier in the course of their illness and this certainly makes sense: the longer someone has been unwell, and the more complex their illness, the less likely they are to respond to any treatment. It seems probable that the longer patients are unwell, the more "stuck" their depression might become. Patients not getting better with many medications might also just have a less 'biological' depression. Something less amenable to physical treatment or medication, their depression persists because of the persistence of unresolved psychological factors or unrelenting relationship or social issues. However, we see many patients who have tried many treatments over the years who do well with TMS, and this is certainly not a good reason to exclude them from trying it. Over the years, I have been pleasantly surprised more times than I care to count, by patients responding when things seemed hopeless. Patients go on to report that they feel better than they have done for years, even decades. TMS treatment is not a panacea for all, the depression of at least one third of patients is untouched by it, but it has now changed the lives of many.

There was also a time when Eileen would have been considered a poor candidate for TMS because of her age. Early studies with TMS suggested that older people responded poorly to this treatment. As we age, our brains tend to shrink. This shrinkage is greatest in the front areas of the brain that we are trying to treat. Therefore, it was proposed that the elderly did not respond to TMS well because the TMS pulse could not reach the "shrunken" frontal brain area that was further from the TMS coil. Fortunately, as the overall strength of the pulses used in TMS treatment has gone up over time, response rates in the elderly seem to have improved and it now seems that elderly patients respond just as well to TMS as younger people do.

After she went home, Eileen and her daughters were extremely pleased that she had returned to normal. She started to help care for her grandchildren again, joined back in with her bridge club, and generally lead a quite active life. She felt like a new woman again. She started to think that she had overcome her depression, that she was finally past it.

This went on without a hiccup for about seven months. Then one day she woke just feeling not quite right. The world seemed bleaker, and it was hard to get out of bed. She really did not want to accept it. After being so well, she refused to accept that the depression might be coming back. She soldiered on for several weeks believing that if she just ignored it, and got on with life, perhaps everything would be OK. This is a frequently too common reaction in patients experiencing a return of depression and one that frequently undermines their capacity to access treatment on a timely basis. For Eileen, unfortunately, this was just wishful thinking. Things gradually worsened. She started having real difficulty getting out of bed in the morning. She stopped calling her family. It was obvious when she saw her psychiatrist that things were not right. She struggled to maintain eye contact, answered questions with one-word answers, and seemed despondent and hopeless. Her psychiatrist said something that surprised her. Why don't you go back and get some more TMS? She had not even thought this possible. She saw herself as having failed treatment: that the return of her depression meant that it had not worked. "Quite the opposite," he said. "Look, you have been great for seven months—go back and do it again!"

So she did. Back for another four weeks of treatment. As is fortunately usually the case with TMS, having worked once, it worked again. Her mood picked up, perhaps even quicker than it did the first time. She was elated and very relieved. However, what would happen now? We discussed several things. First, that even though the antidepressant medication had not really worked all that well for her in the past, it might have a role in stopping the depression from coming back. Antidepressant medication alone, however, may not be all that useful. She could also consider adding lithium to her therapy which can help prevent the return of depression. Understandably given how many medications she had tried over the years, she was reluctant to contemplate taking more drugs now that she was feeling well. Another option was mindfulness-based cognitive therapy which as we discussed in Chapter 2, has been shown to help prevent the return of depression.

Eileen had experienced some mindfulness during her stay in the hospital and was interested in following this up after she went home. She did, however, want to know whether there were any other options, especially whether TMS could be used on an ongoing basis like she had used maintenance ECT in the past. This was possible and certainly something she might want to consider. Although most TMS research has focused on proving that it works when patients are quite depressed, there is some limited evidence that it can be used as a preventative, maintenance approach and many patients are now using it in this way.

However, it is difficult to truly prove that maintenance TMS is effective. To do this adequately, you would need to do a randomized controlled study. Patients who had responded to a course of TMS would need to be randomly given either real TMS or a placebo. If you get the placebo, however, the patients receiving it would be highly likely to realize what they were getting as it would not feel the same as the real treatment they had received previously. This would undermine the trial. So, the evidence we have so far is mainly limited to "open" studies, where patients are aware of the treatment they are receiving. Where controlled trials have been done, they don't mimic the clinical use exactly. For example, a large study conducted in China showed that patients that were provided TMS remained well to a much greater degree than those provided medication, but this study was done in patients who had initially responded to medication, not TMS.

I let Eileen know about these issues, but also a little about our experience. At the time I was treating her, we had been doing maintenance TMS in one form or another for seven or eight years. We had tried two things. One approach was to gradually reduce the intensity of TMS treatment sessions over time. After the course of treatment for depression was finished, patients would initially get one TMS session per week. After a while, this would reduce to one session every second week, then every third week, and then once a month. This approach does seem to work well for some patients and is fairly convenient, but patients commonly seem to get re-emergent symptoms if treatment is too infrequent: providing sessions less than every two weeks often is not enough.

The second approach we have tried we called "clustered maintenance," and this was more commonly used if a patient was accessing TMS as a treatment in the hospital. After discharge from the hospital following a course of TMS, the patient would be readmitted for a weekend about once every four weeks. The patient would receive treatment on a Friday night and two treatments on both Saturday and Sunday. They would get the equivalent of one treatment a week or slightly more, but all in a couple of days. By coming in on the weekend, the patient could keep working or studying. Hopefully, this limited the impact of coming back to the hospital. At the time I treated Eileen we had been doing this type of clustered maintenance for quite some time and so had plenty of experience. I told her that it did not prevent relapse in all of our patients, but it certainly helped most patients stay well longer than they would without it. Some patients had received this sort of maintenance over several years and remained perfectly well, even without medication. At the time of writing this book, we have patients who have now been having maintenance TMS for well over a decade. For many, this has resulted in ongoing stability and an ability to really get back on with their lives without the repeated intrusion of depression. Long-term treatment has not been associated with new or accumulating side effects. Given that Eileen's benefit from TMS was over seven months the first time, I was not convinced that coming in every month was really justified. It makes more sense for patients who only got a couple of months to benefit from TMS.

Another alternative would be for her to use medication and perhaps mindfulness and keep TMS as a type of "rescue treatment" like she had used it on this occasion. That is, to use it if her depression returned despite other treatments. If she was going to do this, I said she should monitor her mood very closely. She should come back for treatment as soon as she felt herself starting to deteriorate. Some patients can do this really well. They keep on top of things and as soon as there is any early sign of relapse, they get treatment to prevent it from getting worse. Sometimes we spend time exploring what usually happens first when they become depressed so that they can get a better idea of what the early signs might be. For some patients, involving their partner or other family members in this can be helpful. Sometimes it is a partner who first notices that things have changed: perhaps that the patient is becoming more irritable or a little bit more withdrawn. The involvement of a family member can also be useful to help overcome some of the resistance to getting treatment. Especially when treatment involves coming back to the hospital, there is often a temptation to try to hope that things will be okay or to hang on as long as possible. Unfortunately, sometimes this means that the depression returns with considerable vengeance before the patient gets treatment again. This can mean a longer and more unpleasant road to recovery.

After all of this discussion, Eileen decided to try mindfulness and to watch and wait as far as the TMS was concerned. She enrolled in a day program that involved attending as an outpatient for eight half days to do a full course of mindfulness based CBT. She also decided to attend an outpatient art therapy group as she had found this very helpful during her hospital stay. She was going to stay on her current medication with the plan to re-attend for TMS should her depression start to come back. She would try to get to treatment early, to prevent a full-blown relapse by intervening early. She discussed this plan with her oldest daughter and her psychiatrist so that they could support her in accessing treatment early should this be required. Hopefully, this would not be for a long time.

Eileen's story, and variants of it, are becoming more and more common. TMS is now becoming a relatively routine part of psychiatric practice in many parts of the world. Since being approved for use in the US it has become quite common, and insurers cover TMS treatment for more than 250 million Americans. There are multiple companies making TMS machines that are approved for clinical use in the US and elsewhere. Machines from the US have been joined by those from Israel, Denmark, the UK, Finland, Russia, Korea, and China. There are an increasing array of technologies to aid TMS delivery. Complex systems to allow targeting based on MRI scans, systems to provide highly custom TMS pulses, and even robots to hold the coil and move it if the patient happens to move their head.

One limitation on the clinical spread of TMS has been the requirement to establish specific infrastructure for its provision. As well as the purchase of equipment, a nurse or similarly trained professional needs to be employed to provide the treatment, and psychiatrists educated in patient assessment and treatment prescription. In some places, TMS services have been set up in individual and small group psychiatric practices but under these circumstances, there may not be sufficient numbers of patients for the service to be viable. Some places provide the treatment as a referral service, for example, in a teaching hospital or university clinic. Patients are referred for treatment and sent back to the referring doctor after the treatment has been provided. This has better scale, but results in the treatment being somewhat divorced from usual care. In other places, entrepreneurial individuals have set up large scale TMS clinics, much like you might see a cosmetic or eye surgery clinic. The most extreme example to date of this is in Tokyo where a large clinic was initially established several years ago with 67 TMS machines, clearly designed to provide a mass market TMS service. Notably, there is a separate VIP entrance for better-healed clientele.

## Theta Burst Stimulation

In 2019, the FDA in the US approved the clinical use of a new TMS protocol referred to as intermittent theta burst stimulation (TBS). TBS was first tested about a decade before this as a way of potentially more potently changing brain activity with TMS pulses. Instead of applying TMS at a single fixed frequency (such as the one or 10 Hz frequencies used typically in depression treatment), TBS involves the application of stimulation at two frequencies mixed together. Specifically, three pulses are applied extremely rapidly, usually 50 times per second (this is referred to as gamma frequency) and these triplets repeated five times per second (this is theta frequency from which the protocol is named). TBS was thought to be a potentially more potent brain stimulation tool as the pattern of pulses would more closely match the way nerve cells fire in the brain.

Research to date has shown that TBS protocols can produce similar effects to standard TMS protocols but in dramatically shorter periods of time: for example 3 minutes instead of 30-40 minutes. A large trial conducted at three hospitals in Canada found no difference in clinical responses to a TBS protocol or standard form of TMS and this data was used in a successful application for FDA approval. This study provides substantial evidence for the effectiveness of TBS, but it is worthy of note that its use has not been supported by the same type of placebo-controlled trials that have supported the use of standard forms of TMS. There also remains unanswered a number of significant questions about how TBS should be best applied to achieve its greatest effects.

Where will TMS fit into psychiatric practice in five or 10 years? It has already become a relatively standard treatment in many places providing a drug free, well tolerated treatment for patients with depression and its use is progressively spreading. Its application is almost completely in patients who have failed to get better with at least one, if not more, medication. What about the significant group of people in our community who just do not want to take medication? There are certainly plenty of these: people who are reluctant to take medication for a whole variety of reasons, some of them very personal and some cultural. I certainly can see a day when some patients would choose to try TMS even before trying medication: some patients will accept the greater inconvenience to be able to avoid commencing drug treatment. It seems highly likely that it will be effective in this group, especially given that TMS is somewhat more effective in patients who are earlier in their illness: we just need the studies to be done to prove it.

The application of TMS is also already expanding in other directions. Much research is underway evaluating its potential use in other psychiatric disorders like schizophrenia, autism, and drug dependence. One TMS system was approved for the treatment of obsessive compulsive disorder in the US in 2019 and use of TMS has even expanded to help people to stop smoking. There are also specific groups of depressed patients where it might prove to be a very useful treatment. For example, depressed pregnant women. Depression in pregnancy is very tricky to treat. If patients are not able to get better with psychotherapy, the options are problematic. There are pregnancy complications associated with the use of the most common antidepressant drugs and it is best to avoid ECT due to the potential impact of the anesthetic and procedure on the pregnancy. Although we have little information as to the impact of a strong magnetic field on the unborn developing baby, very little (probably no) magnetic field from TMS pulse will travel the distance from the surface of the head to the lower abdomen. In fact, the strength of the magnetic field falls away rapidly with distance, such that the exposure of the unborn child is likely to be minimal. In fact, I can imagine that in the future, TMS may prove to be the biological treatment of choice in the future for pregnant women.

Patients who develop depression in their teenage years are also tricky to treat with biological interventions. The most common antidepressants, the serotonin reuptake inhibitors such as fluoxetine (Prozac), have been tested to a limited degree in this age group. There is some evidence that they work but their use is associated with a significant problem. As discussed in Chapter 3, unlike in older people, adolescents treated with antidepressants can experience a significant increase, or even commencement, of suicidal ideation. Clearly, this is not a desirable outcome and one with potentially serious consequences. Insufficient research has evaluated the use of TMS in this age group but certainly, it might prove a valuable treatment option, especially as there is no evidence that TMS use produces increased suicidality.

However, the use of TMS progresses, it is now out of the box and is already changing the treatment of depression. It will be fascinating to see how quickly and widely this happens over the coming years. In the following chapters, we will discuss some other novel treatments developing in the wake of TMS.

## Deep TMS in Depression Treatment

The second clinical device approved for TMS therapy in the US was a so-called deep TMS system made by a company called Brainsway from Israel. This system uses a standard TMS machine but a very different form of TMS coil that produces a magnetic field that is able to pass more deeply into the brain. This field is not necessarily more focused: in fact, to achieve the deeper stimulation, a significantly greater area of the surface of the brain is also stimulated.

Deep TMS was approved for depression following the conduct of a clinical trial that did demonstrate antidepressant activity. However, this trial, and subsequent studies so far have not indicated whether deep TMS is any more, or less, effective than standard forms of TMS.

Brainsway, since the approval of its system for depression, has invested significantly in exploring other potential uses of its deep TMS system. Given the substantial underinvestment of most companies in the field in developing or evaluating new clinical applications, this is a very good thing. In 2019 approval was granted for deep TMS in the treatment of obsessive-compulsive disorder and more recently it has been approved for smoking cessation as well as in the treatment of anxiety in patients with depression. It is likely that further approvals will follow in the coming years.

## 7

# FROM ELECTRIC EELS TO OLYMPIC ATHLETES: TRANSCRANIAL DIRECT CURRENT STIMULATION

TRANSCRANIAL DIRECT CURRENT stimulation (tDCS) is certainly the flavor of the month as far as forms of non-invasive brain stimulation go. Or should I say flavor of the year (or years)? tDCS is a type of brain stimulation that has become so widely used, so widely discussed, and so widely promoted, that is really hard to sort the facts out from the fantasy. If you believe at least some of the publicity, it will make you an Olympic athlete (maybe with a bit of training along the way), boost your memory, enhance your empathy, and cure everything from depression to Parkinson's disease. In this chapter, we will explore what tDCS is, how it works, and whether it is something that is worth considering as a treatment option for depression.

So what is tDCS? It is a relatively simple technique using a weak direct electrical current. Direct means that the current flows in just one direction, unlike the electricity that runs your TV which is alternating, it passes back and forth. This direct current passes between two electrodes that are placed on the scalp. These electrodes are usually contained within two sponges which are soaked in saltwater or some other gel or fluid that conducts electricity. The machines used to generate the electrical signal can be quite simple and even run off a fairly small battery. Someone undergoing a tDCS procedure typically will not feel much at all. They may feel a tickling sensation under the electrodes or an irritating itchy feeling, possibly along with drips of water running out of the electrode pads which have to be quite wet.

The idea of using an electrical current to change brain activity is not new, in fact it is a pretty ancient one. The first documented description of anything like this actually dates all the way back to the Roman empire. In 46AD, Scribonius Largus, physician of the emperor Tiberius, described the use of *torpedos* applied to the head of patients to relieve various ailments: "*The live black torpedo when applied to the painful area relieves and permanently cures some chronic and intolerable protracted headaches . . . carries off pain of arthritis . . . and eases other chronic pains of the body.*"*

The torpedo was not something launched by a Roman version of a submarine but a type of ray, which like an electric eel would produce an electrical discharge or shock. Whilst this was most ingenious, I am not sure the process was subject to any systematic testing or research, let alone regulatory approval!

The notion that electricity could be used for therapeutic purposes was revived several times through the middle ages, For example, in the 11th century, the Muslim physician Ibn-Sidah described the use of torpedo fish to treat what seems to be the condition now considered as epilepsy. However, interest grew considerably with the development of science in the renaissance. In the 1600's in England, William Gilbert, physician to Queen Elizabeth, published *De Magnete*, in which he described the use of electricity in medicine. Gilbert described that when certain materials are rubbed, they will attract light objects. He coined the name "electricity" from the Greek "electron" for amber. During the 1700s the use of electricity for the treatment of paralysis was suggested by Krueger, a Professor of Medicine in Germany and Kratzenstein published a book on electrotherapy. He described a method of treatment, which consisted of seating a patient on a wooden stool, electrifying him by means of a large revolving frictional glass globe, and then drawing sparks from him through the affected body parts.

* *Compositiones Medicae* (46 AD)

The first use of something vaguely resembling modern tDCS came in the early 18th century. After his uncle, Luigi Galvani, invented the first modern DC battery, Giovanni Aldini in Bologna, Italy, used this to treat a patient suffering from "melancholy madness," most likely a form of depression. The patient apparently successfully responded to this therapy over the course of several weeks of treatment.

Forms of tDCS, often called electrotherapy or polarization, increased in popularity, and were used, especially in Europe, well into the 20th century. However, despite the conduct of some scientific experiments and reports, a lack of consistent methods, and consistent results, led to much skepticism, and the field never really flourished.

These approaches died out by 1930 and then had a brief resurgence in the late 1950s-1960s, presumably losing favor again as the use of drugs in psychiatry expanded rapidly. The modern use of tDCS really only dates from 1998 when the first of a series of studies were conducted that more comprehensively explored the effects of tDCS and how it may be potentially applied to alter brain activity. These studies spurred the rapid expansion of interest which remains unabated today.

The main finding of these early reports, and still the foundation of the use of tDCS, was a discovery that there seemed to be quite different effects of tDCS on the brain under each of the two electrodes. These initial studies applied tDCS to the motor cortex, the area of the brain controlling muscles, especially in the hands. This was a quite deliberate choice as the effects of tDCS could be immediately measured. This was done by applying transcranial magnetic stimulation pulses and measuring the size of the muscle twitches that were produced in the hand. A series of pulses would be applied, and the response measured, before and after tDCS was applied to the same site. These initial studies found something really promising: when stimulation was applied with the anode or positive electrode, the muscle twitches produced afterward were larger than before. In contrast, when the effects of stimulation were measured under the cathode (negative electrode) over the motor area, the pulses decreased in size. tDCS appeared to have the capacity to both increase or decrease brain activity, depending on the location and type of the electrode used.

These studies attracted considerable attention and very rapidly, studies started to explore the use of tDCS across both a wider range of stimulation parameters and differing brain areas and functions. There was particular interest in whether tDCS could improve forms of cognitive performance. In fact, tDCS soon became an extraordinarily common tool used in cognitive neuroscience in psychology departments around the world. As the equipment was quite cheap and apparently safe, it was widely adopted as a way of probing brain function. TMS had already been used in this way but the greater cost and complexity of using TMS had limited how widely its use had been adopted.

Scientists were effectively using tDCS to augment the use of neuroimaging technologies in trying to understand the role of different brain regions in specific brain functions. Modern brain imaging tools, especially functional magnetic resonance imaging (fMRI), have been extraordinarily useful tools to demonstrate the involvement of brain regions in specific cognitive functions. However, if brain regions light up on a brain scan during a particular mental task, scientists can only infer that these regions are essential for that behavior, they cannot draw more firm causal inferences. For example, if a number of areas light up in the brain on scanning whilst someone is doing math problems, we cannot know which of these areas are essential to doing math and which are just lighting up for other reasons. It is possible that a particular area lighting up is not critical to the function being examined but this area has been activated for a secondary reason. However, if scientists can then stimulate that area of the brain (with tDCS or TMS) and change its function, this allows much stronger conclusions to be drawn about the relationship between activity in a specific brain area and the brain function being examined.

Researchers also had more ambitious goals. Many were particularly interested in whether tDCS could actually improve cognitive function in a manner that could be applied therapeutically. In this book, we have highlighted some of the considerable limitations that there are with existing treatments for depression. However, the current state of treatments available for cognitive disorders make it seemed like we have an excess of riches in the availability of treatment for problems of mood. Frankly, we have minimal capacity with drugs to meaningfully change cognitive disorders. There are a small number of drugs available for Alzheimer's disease but these at best only subtly delay the progression of the cognitive problems produced by this disorder. Problems of cognition also affect patients with a range of other disorders such as Parkinson's disease and schizophrenia and we really have no effective therapy for these issues.

In this context, is not surprising that there has been considerable excitement about the possibility that tDCS could be developed as an effective and safe therapy. Studies have exploded exploring whether tDCS can improve thinking abilities ranging from different types of memory through to the ability to excel at math. There has been much excitement at the results of some of these studies, even though most of the research studies have only tested short-term effects in healthy individuals, not patients with cognitive disorders. In fact, most studies have only shown benefits over minutes, not really the time scale that is clinically useful.

The idea that we may be able to improve thinking has also caught the imagination of the public far more widely, from entrepreneurs to individuals wanting to "hack" their own brains. Plans have been posted on the internet describing how to build a tDCS device at home and companies have sprung up selling these devices directly to the public for self-use. Generally, these self-use indications have not been for the treatment of medical conditions. The proposed applications have included claims to improve the performance of users playing video games, to improve academic or general thinking ability and in one more notable commercial application, to improve sporting performance. In regard to the later, the company Halo Neuroscience was established to develop and market a tDCS device providing stimulation to the motor systems of the brain and has been heavily marketed using case studies of prominent Olympic and professional athletes.

There are two major problems with these home use applications. First, in most cases they are supported by little or no evidence that the device will produce the effects that they are being proposed to do. In one notable example, the "focus" tDCS device was promoted as improving a wide range of cognitive functions well before there was evidence to support these claims. The first independent academic study exploring the claims of cognitive improvement with this device actually found the opposite: evidence of temporary cognitive impairment on a specific task. It is not possible to read the academic studies suggesting evidence of cognitive improvement and assume that these commercially available devices will produce similar effects. The systems are too different, for example, in the types of electrodes used, often optimized for useability, not effectiveness, to make this assumption.

There is also a second, even bigger, issue. At this stage, we have limited evidence that long-term use is actually safe. Research exploring the safety of tDCS has been limited to weeks, not the months or years that some of these non-medical applications propose that its use might be extended for. There is also minimal evidence of safety in special populations that might be vulnerable to marketing claims. Stimulant drugs, amphetamines, and related compounds are commonly used by adolescents to improve their capacity to study and perform in competitive exams. It is a very small leap to assume tDCS might become widely used in much the same way despite the lack of evidence showing long-term safety in this age group. Even if it is only a small group who starts to use the technology in this way, it will create competitive pressure for others to follow suit. This already seems to have started. In 2017 NPR reported that sales of certain tDCS devices were peaking around college midterms and finals.*

These problems have become prominent because non-medical uses of tDCS devices are restricted by few regulations and the barriers to the development of these devices are made low by the simplicity of the technology. In many countries, there are no restrictions on the capacity of companies to market devices to the public as long as they are not making claims of effectiveness in a medical disorder. It is fine to sell the device to improve your thinking if you are considered "healthy" but not if you have something like Alzheimer's disease.

In recent years, there has emerged a potentially even greater concern about the use of tDCS, something that could apply to all of its uses. Does it work at all?

---

* https://www.npr.org/sections/alltechconsidered/2017/01/07/507133313/ students-zap-their-brains-for-a-boost-for-better-or-worse

This concern initially arose in about the most basic application of tDCS, the studies showing increases and decreases in activity in the motor cortex or muscle area of the brain: the type of studies that initially revived interest in tDCS. In 2014, researchers from the University of Melbourne published a meta-analysis of these studies: an analysis of the effects of all the studies exploring the use of tDCS published until that time. The results gathered considerable attention, with the headline writers of New Scientist wondering "*Has the brain-zap backlash begun?*"* The paper essentially said that tDCS seems to produce some subtle effects on one measure of brain activity but nothing on most of the measures analyzed. This seemed to reflect what other researchers had increasingly been seeing. It was often possible to show some group effects (that is, across a group of people studied, an effect might be seen) but for individual subjects, the effects of tDCS could vary a lot. Anodal tDCS might increase brain activity in some subjects as expected, other individuals would show no change, and the opposite effects might be seen. The overall effects were just not reliable or predictable.

A second study published by the same authors 2 years later had a similar impact, although was also controversial. The second paper applied the same methods to test whether tDCS had effects on cognitive functions (types of thinking), something that many other research groups are quite invested in. The study analyzed the results from 400 separate studies. This seems an impressive number: conclusions drawn from large samples are usually the most reliable. However, the approach adopted in this study has been widely criticized, for quite substantial and important reasons. The main problem was that the paper included studies using tDCS to try and improve many different types of cognition. There were actually only a small number of studies on each type of cognition, undermining the strength of the results. Oxford neuroscientist Roi Cohen Kadosh was quoted in New Scientist as saying, "*it is very premature to do what they did. They did have a large sample size, but they fractured it so that they are comparing the results of three or four studies*

* https://www.newscientist.com/article/dn26636-has-the-brain-zap-backlash-begun/

*and expecting to see something meaningful. It's the easiest thing in science to not find results."\**

The debate on the degree of the effects seen in these studies has continued. Further meta-analyses have shown that tDCS may improve working memory, the ability to hold information in mind, which is considered an important building block for other aspects of thinking. This is one area of thinking about which there is a reasonably large collection of studies and we can be more confident about the results.

In relation to the use of tDCS as a clinical tool to improve cognition, or by gamers or college students studying for exams, the main problem is not the analyses, it is the studies they are analyzing. The vast majority of this research has just explored very short-term effects of tDCS on thinking. Most researchers have looked for these effects in the first 30 or 60 minutes after a single short session of stimulation. How these effects translate to the potential long-term therapeutic use of repeatedly stimulating your brain over time, is often completely unclear.

This brings us back to depression. Does tDCS have any use in its treatment? This is a question that has attracted interest since not long after tDCS was rediscovered at the end of the 1980s. The first clinical study testing tDCS in depressed patients was published in 2006 reporting the treatment of ten patients who each received five days of either active tDCS or a sham. Antidepressant effects were reported which has stimulated multiple attempts to expand on this research over the years since. Some of these studies have reported effects that are greater than placebo, or similar to the effects seen with medication, but there have also been studies that have failed to find benefits of tDCS stimulation. Notably, several of the negative studies have been in groups of patients with more treatment resistant forms of depression.

A group of Brazilian researchers have conducted an important series of studies. They initially showed that combining tDCS and an antidepressant medication seemed to produce greater effects than the tDCS or drug therapy alone. However, they then conducted a much larger study directly comparing a common antidepressant, escitalopram, with

\* https://www.newscientist.com/article/dn26874-second-blow-to-the-head-for-effects-of-brain-zapping/#ixzz6Eehvk800

tDCS in 245 depressed patients: importantly these were not medication resistant patients. TDCS was superior to the placebo but was not as effective as the medication therapy.

There have now been almost as many meta-analyses pooling the results of tDCS studies as there have been individual studies themselves. Most of these have found some benefits of tDCS compared to sham or placebo stimulation although at least one found no difference in response and remission rates which are more important ways of judging whether treatment is effective than the measures adopted in a number of the other analyses.

## What Measures Are Used to Judge Effectiveness?

As described earlier, the degree of depression experienced by patients is usually assessed with standard questionnaires which produce a numerical score. If this score comes down with treatment, it indicates that symptoms are improving. Many studies take these numerical scores and assess whether the overall reductions achieved with the new treatment, in this case tDCS, are greater than the reductions seen with placebo therapy. This approach can demonstrate a benefit (for example an average 15% reduction might be better than a 5% reduction) but the treatment might not be producing clinically helpful effects.

An alternative approach is to compare response or even better, remission rates. Response rates usually refer to the number of patients who have shown a reduction of depression scores by at least 50%, a halving of the depression level. Remission usually means that a patient's score drops to a level where they are reporting minimal or no symptoms. If a new therapy produces a meaningful remission rate, and this is substantially more than placebo, this gives a lot more confidence that it is likely to be useful in clinical practice. In one tDCS meta-analysis, the treatment produced a 12.2% remission rate, compared to 5.4% for placebo: this was statistically significant but does not seem all that clinically meaningful.*

* Berlim M.T., Van den Eynde F., Daskalakis Z.J. Clinical utility of transcranial direct current stimulation (tDCS) for treating major depression: A systematic review and meta-analysis of randomized, double-blind and sham-controlled trials. J. Psychiatr. Res. 2013; 47:1–7. DOI: 10.1016/j.jpsychires.2012.09.025

This is all a little disappointing. tDCS, at least how it has been used to date, seems to have antidepressant effects, but they appear to be fairly weak and not very consistent across patients, even when used in patients not considered treatment resistant. In contrast, a lot of the research establishing the effectiveness of TMS has been conducted in more challenging treatment resistant patients.

Could tDCS have a role still? This is possible. There are still things that may be done to improve the application of tDCS although there are relatively few features of the technique that are amenable to improvement. I would like to tell you a little bit about another patient of mine whose story suggests the possibility of an interesting, if somewhat niche, place in therapy.

Brian was 48 when I first considered using tDCS in his care, but he had been in psychiatric treatment for almost 20 years. He first experienced depression in his early 20s, responding well to the SSRI fluoxetine. He stopped this after about six months and remained well until his depression returned at age 28. His second episode also responded well to fluoxetine, this time he stayed on it for a little longer but came off again after about a year. His third episode followed a redundancy from work when he was 35. He was tried on fluoxetine, this time without success, followed by trials of venlafaxine, mirtazapine, and sertraline. He saw a new psychiatrist the next year who tried him on several other antidepressants as well as several antipsychotics. He saw two psychologists: with one he did a course of CBT. None of this helped. His second psychiatrist then referred him for a course of TMS. This was done over four weeks as an inpatient and was a resounding success. His depression resolved fully, and he went home, happy and looking forward to reengaging in life.

The relief was short lived. Within about six weeks his sense of gloom and darkness started to return. Anxious and fearful of a full relapse, he came back to the hospital, wanting further TMS. He had these ten sessions over two weeks and responded again, fully. He went home the second time requesting maintenance TMS and was booked to come back for clustered maintenance, with a plan for 5 treatments every four weeks. This went well for quite a few months; he was stable between treatments and returned to work. But this did not last. After a while, his improved mood was not persisting for the full four weeks. The last few days before the next round of treatment he would really struggle. Initially the five sessions would be enough for him to bounce back but gradually the length of time he felt well shrank and the duration of TMS required to get him back on track lengthened: soon he was often having ten sessions instead of five.

Eventually, a decision was reluctantly made to reduce the interval between his treatments to only three weeks, and at times, he even seemed to need it every two. With this he was much better, his mood normal almost all of the time. However, every attempt to stretch the time out between sessions failed. He continued on like this for several years. We tried a variety of different medications including lithium to see if these would help stave off the return of symptoms, but none made any difference. He could remain well, but at a real cost: the frequency of treatment sessions was really intrusive on his work and family life.

One day I came up with a suggestion out of left field. Why don't we think about tDCS. I was not thinking about replacing TMS with tDCS. I was thinking about trying this as an addition: could he try and use tDCS on a regular basis between the TMS sessions to see if this would provide some additional benefit and enable him to have to come back for TMS less frequently? This was not really a suggestion based on science but a hope that we could come up with something that could solve the puzzle of his predicament: that TMS was effective in treating his depression and even keeping him well, but it was really impractical for him to have frequent enough TMS to stay well in the long-term. There were two options to do this, only one practical. There was at the time, one tDCS machine available on the market in Australia and approved for use in the treatment of depression. I would need to spend $6,000 or so to purchase the device and Brian would have to come to the hospital on a regular basis to receive treatment, just like TMS: not really a practical improvement. There was also no way for him to claim reimbursement for the cost of this treatment.

The second option was more practical but more out of the mainstream. Brian would go online, and purchase a "direct to consumer" non-clinical tDCS machine, I would show him how to use it for the treatment of depression and he would then apply treatment himself at home on an ongoing basis. This would give him the capacity to continue the treatment on an ongoing basis, in between his regular TMS. Hopefully adding the tDCS would allow him to reduce how frequently he would need to come to the hospital. However, he would be using an unregulated device and I could in no way guarantee the quality of what he would be using. It was uncomfortable ground to be proposing this, more like snake oil than sensible medicine. But even still, it seemed like the most reasonable option amongst a sea of bad ones.

Brian actually jumped at the chance to try this. I think he would have jumped at the opportunity to try anything that might reduce how frequently he was having to come to the hospital. I gave him the website for a tDCS machine which seemed reasonable, it cost him about $500 with a little more for some bottles of saline to soak the electrodes. Once it had been delivered, he came back to see me, and brought the device, and his wife, along: I had told him he was going to need a helper to put the electrodes on. We took out the various straps and I set them up so the positive electrode was positioned over the left frontal part of his brain and the second electrode was positioned above his right eye. This is the arrangement that has been used in most of the trials of tDCS in depression. I wrote out a series of instructions for his wife, she took some photos to help her remember the set up and we marked the straps to help her as well. Next, I wrote out a plan for how he was going to use the tDCS: for the first few weeks he would do one session a day, for 20 minutes, with a 1 milliamp current. We would first check if he was tolerating this without an issue and then explore whether it would have an effect on his need for TMS or if the dose needed to be higher.

Over the next couple of months, we adjusted Brian's routine and began to see that yes, it was making a difference. After about six weeks of daily sessions, we settled on him doing three sessions a week, still 20 minutes in length but at a 1.5 milliamp current. He would sometimes notice an annoying irritation under the electrodes but had no other side effects. After two months he was able to get through three weeks between TMS sessions without any sign of his depression returning and a few months later, he successfully increased the interval to four weeks. At the time of writing, we are planning to see if the TMS can be stretched out further: to five, then six weeks, hopefully to every two or three months.

This is clearly not a typical or evidence-based use of tDCS and was only considered out of a degree of therapeutic desperation. I do not know yet how long the benefits will last or how intensively we should continue the tDCS long-term. We will try to reduce how frequently Brian does the tDCS sessions but for now, both he and his wife are keen to continue as it is.

I am by no means advocating for this type of use of tDCS, but given the potential for its home application, studies should further explore its use as a maintenance treatment approach. To date, this type of application has not been the subject of much research. Some studies have used maintenance tDCS and there is a suggestion that how commonly the sessions are used (for example once or twice per week) does relate to how effective it is likely to be at preventing the return of depression. At this stage though, we really have no idea of what the ideal schedule might be and how much this might need to vary between patients.

So, what place does tDCS currently have? Answering this remains confused by differing regulatory environments and the lack of a single clear standard on which to judge the evidence of effectiveness. The studies conducted to date suggest that tDCS has antidepressant effects but the evidence is limited and the strength of effects much less than that seen with TMS. tDCS devices have been approved for use in some countries, but notably not in systems where approval is dependent on a rigorous evaluation of evidence of effectiveness or broader assessment of value such as whether tDCS therapy is cost effective.

Clearly as illustrated by the case of Brian, I have "voted with my feet" adopting its use to a limited degree. My clinical practice is unusual, however, in the type of patients I treat, and often in their interest in exploring novel, unproven options. In Brian's case, we only progressed after a lengthy discussion of how unknown the risks and benefits were, a discussion that involved his wife as well. I would not have been comfortable going down this path unless I felt he had a really good understanding of how little we knew about what he was getting himself into.

This situation may well change very quickly. As I suggested at the start, there is a considerable body of tDCS research underway. This may establish the evidence justifying its more widespread therapeutic use but for now, we will have to wait. One approach to potentially improve the clinical effects seen with tDCS, which my research group has pioneered, is to combine stimulation with some sort of activity that results in the targeted area of the brain being 'activated' more naturally. For example, if we are targeting frontal cognitive areas of the brain with tDCS, having the patient engage in challenging cognitive problems to intrinsically activate that area of the brain at the same time. This approach seems to make a lot of sense. As I said before, anodal tDCS does not make nerve cells fire but increases the likelihood that they will. Therefore, if we can stimulate and activate the same area of the brain, this should produce greater nerve cell firing which hopefully will then embed some change over time in the activity of that region with therapeutic value. We have conducted preliminary studies showing that this appears to be the case but there is still a lot of research to go into proving that this can make a big enough difference for tDCS to be clinically useful.

One aspect that lessens my overall enthusiasm for tDCS is the overall limitations of the technique. Unlike TMS, where we have the capacity to increasingly personalize and make more specific a variety of aspects of the technology (such as the pulse strength, the frequency, the location of stimulation), there seems only limited capacity to improve the application of tDCS. Increasing the current strength much beyond 2 milliamps, as is now commonly used, produces increasing skin irritation. Considerable research has focused on making the electrode positions more specific, but this is only a limited advance. There is not much else that is likely to improve tDCS application to any substantial degree.

There are, however, some tDCS related techniques that might just have even greater potential. Part of the problem with tDCS is that it just involves a simple, fixed, one way electrical current. There are several limitations that arise from this. First, it is possible that the brain will adapt to a fixed current. As the tDCS current changes slightly the electrical charge around superficial neurons in the brain, the brain's homeostatic processes, which work to keep everything in balance, might just correct this effect, limiting the overall impact of the stimulation itself. *Random noise stimulation* has been proposed as a way to address this. This involves applying a similar electrical current but randomly varying the strength of the current over time. The current can have the element of a direct current—that is, all the current goes in the same direction but with variable strength—or randomly vary in the direction as well (so it passes back and forth between the two electrodes). Some studies have started to explore the use of random noise stimulation, but its potential is far from established and there has been minimal use of it in the therapy of any disorders.

There is a type of stimulation that already has some early clinical support and also seemingly addresses the second major limitation with tDCS: the lack of any capacity to personalize the stimulation parameters. This is called *transcranial alternating current stimulation* (tACS). As the title says, the current alternates—goes back and forth—instead of in just one direction. tACS is proposed to work in a quite different way from tDCS: through interaction with the intrinsic electrical activity of the brain.

Although people often talk about the chemical neurotransmitters in the brain, the fundamental language of the brain is much more electrical than chemical. Nerve cells do not typically fire by themselves but in groups. Their firing is also not random. They tend to fire repeatedly in certain patterns. The frequency of their activity is the number of times that a group of nerve cells fires per second. Nerve cells in different areas of the brain tend to communicate through this coordinated firing at specific frequencies: two brain areas that are apparently interacting will be firing at the same frequency and usually "in phase"—firing and then resting at the same time. These coordinated firings are called *oscillations*.

These electrical signals can be recorded with electrical sensors placed on the scalp; a process called electroencephalography (EEG). EEG is most commonly used to diagnose epilepsy where there are abnormal patterns of electrical activity associated with the seizures caused by this condition. EEG can also be used to study brain activity. There are clear patterns of activity commonly seen on EEG recordings (see box on the next page) and we increasingly understand the role of activity at these specific frequencies in different areas of the brain.

**Common Patterns of Activity Recorded with EEG**

- **Delta:** 0.5-3Hz, usually prominent in sleep
- **Theta:** 4-8Hz, prominent in deep relaxation
- **Alpha:** 8-15Hz, increases during relaxation or passive attention
- **Beta:** 12-35Hz, increases during external attention
- **Gamma:** 35-80Hz, prominent in effortful cognitive activity

One of the most fascinating findings regarding brain oscillations is their relationship to working memory. As mentioned earlier, working memory is the capacity to keep information in mind, over relatively short periods of time. It is possible to test working memory by getting subjects to remember simple lists, for example, of numbers, letters, objects, or words. The number of items that can reliably be remembered will differ between people. If we measure EEG during this type of activity, we see an interesting pattern. First, doing this seems to stimulate activity in several frequencies and different brain areas including alpha activity, theta, and gamma. The most striking effect though, is that the number of items that an individual will remember directly relates to the number of fast gamma waves that happen within the timespan of each slow theta wave. If there are seven gamma waves for each theta wave, the individual will remember seven items, if there are eight, they will remember eight, and so on. The relationship between these theta and gamma waves seems somehow related to the encoding of this information in memory.

This observation has led to a fairly natural extension, is it possible to manipulate activity at one or other of these frequencies to try and change working memory, potentially improve it? There seem to be two ways you could increase the number of gamma waves within its theta cycle: you could either speed up gamma activity so more would fit in a fixed theta wave, or you could slow down the theta activity itself. Researchers have started exploring these approaches using tACS. tACS can potentially be applied at a slower theta frequency or a faster gamma frequency than is usually displayed by an individual subject. Early research has suggested that it is possible to do this in the short term: it will be a bigger challenge to prove that these effects last and can be used as a treatment approach to enhance working memory.

If tDCS works by changing the likelihood of nerve cells firing, is this the case for tACS? For a start, there is no positive or negative electrode when doing tACS as the current flows back and forth between both. Therefore, we should not expect a change in the excitability of the brain under the electrodes as you do with tDCS, and this is not seen in tACS experiments. tACS does produce an important, different, effect: *entrainment*. Entrainment is a process whereby the intrinsic rhythms of the brain become synchronized with a form of external stimulation, in this case, the tACS current. For example, if tACS is applied at the alpha rhythm of 10Hz, nerve cells in the areas stimulated will increasingly fire at 10Hz, in synchrony with the external stimulation. When the tACS finishes, this entrained activity will continue for some time: not usually a long time after a single period of stimulation but presumably more and more if stimulation is repeated over time. Even when the entrainment has not continued, there are measurable effects on brain activity: it is like the entrainment acts as a trigger for other brain changes.

There is an interesting feature of entrainment that suggests that tACS is a technique that ideally should be specifically tuned for each individual subject or patient. Within each frequency band, for example, the alpha band, it is possible to detect a "peak frequency" of activation that will differ between people. This is the specific frequency within the band that an individual subject's brain tends to oscillate at during the particular circumstances they are under (for example at rest and or during a specific thinking activity). For example, nerves in my brain might oscillate at the alpha rhythm of 9.7Hz when I am resting with my eyes closed. This type of peak frequency can be measured and assessed with EEG.

Getting back to tACS and entrainment. Entrainment is most likely to occur when stimulation is applied close to the peak frequency for an individual person (see box on the next page). Specifically, a weaker current will be required to induce entrainment the closer the stimulation frequency is to the subject's own frequency. So for me, trying to entrain my alpha rhythms would be far more effective if stimulations would be applied at close to, or exactly at, 9.7Hz. For someone else, this could be 10.3Hz, 8.9Hz, etc. Individually tuning the tACS would seem to be the most effective way to produce changes in relevant types of brain activity with tACS. The stimulation frequency applied could then be continued at the same frequency or be gradually modified, up or down, to try and shift the pattern of oscillations for an individual subject. To date, however, most of the initial tACS research has only used fixed frequencies, for example, 10 Hz in everybody. Therefore, we will need to wait a bit longer to see the real potential of tACS.

### Arnold Tongue and tACS

Arnold Tongue is a mathematical concept named after an important 20th century Russian Mathematician, Vladimir Arnold, which has been adapted to the principles of tACS and entrainment. In the context of tACS, this refers to the idea that it will be "easier" to entrain brain oscillations with an external stimulus, in this case, tACS, when the external frequency is as close as possible to the intrinsic oscillatory frequency for an individual person. More precisely, the closer the external frequency is to the internal frequency, the lower the power or amplitude of the stimulation that will be required to produce entrainment. For example, if my individual alpha frequency is 9.5Hz, it will take a weaker tACS signal to induce entrainment if stimulation is applied at 9.6Hz than at 10.6Hz. This indicates that there is considerable potential to optimize some applications of tACS by individualization of the stimulation frequency through the measurement of this prior to the application of stimulation.

Is there any evidence that tACS can have therapeutic effects? Although it is very early days in this research, the answer is yes. Studies are far less advanced than in some of the other areas we have discussed but the preliminary impression is good. There are early studies showing that appropriately targeted tACS might have value in reducing the hallucinations (voices) or separately the negative symptoms (problems with motivation, ability to experience pleasure, slowness of thinking) experienced by people with schizophrenia, and there are case reports of benefits of tACS in obsessive compulsive disorder. In regard to treating depression, the first study using tACS came out in 2019.* Only 5 days of treatment was provided but this was sufficient to show antidepressant effects, with alpha frequency (10Hz) stimulation more so than gamma (40Hz). Individualizing frequency, which I have suggested is likely to have more potent effects, has not been explored yet. However, the initial evidence looks promising and I look forward to seeing the results of the studies that will come out over the coming years testing this out.

tDCS, tRNS, and tACS may not be the end of the exploration of non-invasive electrical brain stimulation. Studies are already testing a new approach, transcranial pulsed direct current stimulation, a cross between tDCS and tACS. There is also an interesting approach in development that combines multiple frequencies of alternating current stimulation in a method designed to get stimulation deep into the brain. This would be a major breakthrough: all of the non-invasive approaches developed so far can only stimulate relatively superficial brain regions. Stimulating deeper stimulation, without the necessity of an invasive procedure, would be very novel. However, in Chapter 9, we will explore what might actually be possible with deeper stimulation, but of a much more invasive type.

---

* Double-blind, randomized pilot clinical trial targeting alpha oscillations with transcranial alternating current stimulation (tACS) for the treatment of major depressive disorder (MDD) Morgan L. Alexander, Sankaraleengam Alagapan, Courtney E. Lugo, Juliann M. Mellin, Caroline Lustenberger, David R. Rubinow & Flavio Fröhlich, Translational Psychiatry volume 9, Article number: 106 (2019)

## 8

# BRIGHT LIGHT THERAPY AND DEPRESSION TREATMENT

IN THIS CHAPTER we will explore an area that is rather marginal to the mainstream treatment of depression in most places, but as you will read, not deservedly so. I refer here to the use of light therapy in the treatment of various types of depression. This is an approach for which there is a quite reasonable and growing body of evidence, but one which has remained very much in the shadows. This has presumably resulted from the absence of strong financial incentives to introduce light therapy widely into clinical practice. Business models and clear pathways which incentivize prescribing doctors do not necessarily result from the development of a straightforward treatment such as this.

So what is light therapy, or more appropriately termed, bright light therapy or BLT? It is the use of a very bright light, administered to a patient through a lamp, lightbox, or even goggles, for a specific period of time and importantly at a very specific time of day. Before we explore the use of BLT and how it might be effective, it is worth spending a short time exploring some aspects of the history of the use of light in medicine, as although BLT is a modern treatment, it has ancient antecedents.

These antecedents are genuinely old and involve that most classical of ancient medical figures, Hippocrates himself. Around 400 BC Hippocrates described Heliotherapy, the use of sunshine in the treatment of problems of mood and mental health. He was especially interested in the effects that seasons of the year could have on health, as well as the orientation of ones living space in regard to the sun. These ideas continued with the writings of Roman doctors such as Galen and then perhaps most clearly by Aretaeus of Cappadocia. Aretaeus was a prominent Greek physician who lived in a region of what is modern day Turkey, in the first century. In a series of eight classical medical texts, Aretaeus described a series of diseases outlining their classical characteristics. Within his writings on mental disorders, he described hysteria, mania, and melancholy. In fact, he was the first writer to link the latter two conditions, developing the idea of what is now considered a bipolar disorder. Even more impressively, in the context of this chapter, was his formulation of treatment: *"Lethargics are to be laid in the light, and exposed to the rays of the sun (for the disease is gloom)."*

From the Greeks and Romans, we can jump forward to the early 19th century. Jean-Étienne Dominique Esquirol worked at the famous Salpêtrière Hospital in Paris from 1799 onwards, initially as a student of Philippe Pinel, one of the most influential early pioneers of compassionate mental health care and the developer of "moral therapy." Esquirol studied the conditions in asylums throughout France and reported back to the government, strongly arguing for the reform of facilities, especially those outside of Paris. He argued the need for the "medicalization" of the treatment of the "insane" and the need for the treatment of patients in specialist hospitals to be led by specialist trained physicians. In regard to our topic here, he proposed that "a lunatic hospital is an instrument of cure." He argued that the physical design of hospitals should support the care of patients and that there are specific elements of the design of hospitals that should be implemented to improve the outcomes of patients. A critical design element was maximizing the exposure of patients to light. This principle influenced the development of a series of hospitals throughout France during the first decades of the 19th century.

The next big development in the use of light as a part of medical care, although not prominently in the treatment of disorders of mental health, came about at the end of the 19th century. It was actually in the treatment of tuberculosis where helio (sunlight) therapy became extremely popular. Sanatoria were increasingly built in country areas, for the treatment of patients with tuberculosis, with the movement catalyzed in Switzerland. Around the same time, the Danish physicist Niels Ryberg Finsen, a future Nobel prize winner, developed the first lamp capable of producing ultraviolet rays. This was adopted in medicine in the treatment of Lupus Vulgaris, a tuberculosis infection of the skin.

We finally reconnect light treatment and mental health in the mid-1980s. In 1984, Norman Rosenthal and colleagues published the first description of seasonal affective disorder (SAD). The aptly named SAD is a condition where patients experience periods of depression during the darker, colder months of winter and fall with resolution in spring and summer. It appears to be more common in countries further from the equator as may be expected given the shorter days and less intense sunlight, especially in winter.

From this first description of SAD, Rosenthal moved quite quickly to testing the use of light therapy as a treatment for SAD. He described the first series of patients with SAD treated with a light lamp, reporting promising clinical benefits. Specifically, patients were treated with exposure to fluorescent light, providing light across the light spectrum, for three hours at dawn and three hours at dusk. This treatment, repeated daily for two weeks, produced substantial antidepressant effects.

Since 1984, the methods of the provision of what has become known as Bright Light Therapy (BLT) have gradually evolved. The standard approach in use now typically involves a daily 30 minute treatment session which is much more convenient than the original approach. The light provided is typically full spectrum visible light at an intensity of 10,000 Lux, quite a strong light. Treatment is undertaken first thing in the morning and the light is positioned so that the patient is not looking directly at the light source, but a considerable amount of the light will pass onto the retina at the back of the eye.

Given the specific reason for its development, it is not surprising that the major focus of interest in the development of BLT has been in the treatment of SAD. A series of clinical trials have been conducted over the last couple of decades although these have been relatively modest in overall size. Generally speaking, these trials have indicated that BLT does have a significant therapeutic benefit in patients with SAD although there is far less convincing evidence that BLT can actually prevent the development of an episode of seasonal depression. Importantly, the degree of therapeutic benefit achieved in individual patients with BLT treatment is substantial and clinically meaningful. Studies have shown that a significant proportion of patients receiving this treatment will have a complete, or almost complete, resolution of depressive symptoms. This is not just a treatment of results in a small reduction in symptoms, making people feel a little bit better: it can make a sizeable and consequential difference.

Although, as we have addressed so far, the focus of use with BLT has been in patients with SAD, there has also been interest in its possible use for patients with more standard forms of depression, those without seasonal variability. In this context, clinical trials have been conducted evaluating the addition of BLT as a standalone treatment or the effects of BLT provided in addition to standard antidepressant medication treatment of depression. The studies conducted to date have been criticized by some due to the relatively small groups of patients included and the challenges of providing adequate placebo treatment. However, the results of the trials appear to be relatively consistent: BLT appears to produce antidepressant effects that are similar to the therapeutic benefits achieved with antidepressant medication. In addition, the provision of BLT plus medication appears to produce greater benefits than medication alone. For example, one trial compared treatment with the antidepressant venlafaxine to the combination of BLT plus venlafaxine in a group of significantly depressed inpatients with depression. 76% of patients receiving the combination therapy, compared to 24% on medication alone, achieved the predefined improvement in depression scores considered a meaningful clinical benefit.*

In addition to these trials, a number of studies have investigated the use of BLT in specific populations of patients with depression. For example, one study demonstrated significant antidepressant effects in women with depression who were pregnant and a second study found benefits of BLT in adolescent patients with depression, a group for which

* Pınar Güzel Özdemir, Murat Boysan, Michael H Smolensky, Yavuz Selvi, Adem Aydin, Ekrem Yilmazo. Comparison of venlafaxine alone versus venlafaxine plus bright light therapy combination for severe major depressive disorder. J Clin Psychiatry 2015 May;76(5): e645-54. doi: 10.4088/JCP.14m09376.

there are few proven therapeutic options. There is also some evidence of therapeutic benefits of BLT in patients with depression who have bipolar disorder although the outcome of studies in this condition have not been as consistent.

Given these fairly consistent findings, is worth asking how this could work, especially if we are considering the use of BLT in non-seasonal depression. One thing we do know is that there is a clear pathway for the effect of light to influence brain function. In the retinas at the back of our eyes, there are specific proteins whose role is in the detection of the intensity of light, as well as the standard rods and cones that many people are aware of that help us perceive color. Stimulation of this light intensity detecting protein (called melanopsin) triggers specific nerve cells to send signals deep into the brain. These nerve cells connect to centers of the brain responsible for biological rhythms such as our sleep–wake cycle and the production of important hormones such as melatonin, which many people take in tablet form to help with sleep. It is thought that BLT may help patients with SAD by resetting or modifying some of these biological clocks but also that it could also have benefits through effects on serotonin, the brain chemical we explored in a previous chapter.

If BLT can be effective, what is the downside? Actually, the side effects of BLT are relatively mild compared to issues that can arise with antidepressant medication. The most common problems that can occur are typically headaches, eyestrain, or nausea. There are some eye and medical conditions that would warrant careful specialist review by an ophthalmologist or other expert, before the commencement of treatment. Interestingly, and consistent with all established antidepressant treatments, there are three reports in the literature of BLT resulting in patients with bipolar disorder experiencing a switch from depression to a manic state.

Given the impressive safety profile, and emerging evidence supporting the use of BLT in SAD and depression itself, why is this treatment not more widely used? Although a small number of insurers in the US may reimburse the cost of light boxes for SAD, this is certainly not widespread, and BLT is not funded in most jurisdictions around the world.

However, the equipment for the provision of BLT is really not that prohibitively expensive: clinically tested devices are available on the Internet for less than $200. It is perhaps the simplicity of this technology that has somewhat paradoxically limited the uptake of this approach. Given that no one company has a monopoly on the sale of these devices, there is no incentive for a company to invest heavily in achieving clinical or funding approval. There are also no clear "incentives" to drive doctors to adopt this sort of approach: they are not reimbursed for the prescription of, or supervision of BLT treatment outside of regular consultation fees. They are also not bombarded with advertising like they are for the latest and "greatest" drug that has come on the market. The use of this treatment seems as likely to be driven by the interest of educated patients than by the mental health professionals involved in their care. For patients with any degree of seasonality in depressive symptoms, and perhaps patients with depression more broadly including those who wish to avoid medication treatment, BLT certainly should be a treatment consideration.

# 9

# DEEP BRAIN STIMULATION

JANE WAS 54 years old when she was first referred to me for assessment. By this time, she had already lived several interesting lives. She began by raising a large family of 5 children on a rural property in the country of South Australia. As her children grew older, Jane returned to study, obtained qualifications in real estate marketing, and then returned to full-time work. All of this came to a halt when she first developed depression, the illness striking in her mid-40s, seemingly out of the blue.

Jane gradually became increasingly withdrawn, unmotivated, lethargic, and sad. She began to think that life was just too hard and saw suicide as a realistic and sensible way out. She struggled to even get out of bed in the morning, and if she could have, she would have stayed there all day long. Her family became increasingly worried, ultimately taking her to see the local family doctor. He diagnosed her with depression and prescribed fluoxetine or Prozac, probably the most widely prescribed of any of the anti-depressant medications at the time.

The fluoxetine provided some transient relief but as happens all too frequently with antidepressant medications, the beneficial effects wore off over a matter of months. She was tried on a second medication again with limited effect and then referred to see a psychiatrist. Over the next two years, Jane's life was a blur of medications and therapy. She tried drug after drug. Some of these gave her a brief period of relief, but more caused debilitating side effects. Nausea, dizziness, insomnia, and lethargy to name a few. She saw several psychologists for cognitive behavioral therapy and interpersonal therapy: talking therapies that encouraged her to focus on potentially harmful negative thoughts and problems in her relationships. None of this made a lot of sense to her and it certainly did not lift the black veil of depression. She became even more withdrawn from life, only seeing family and friends when she really had to. In turn, her family became increasingly worried: this was not the vibrant mother, wife, aunty, or friend that they had known.

Her doctors became increasingly desperate. Combinations of antidepressant medications were tried: taking more than one medication at a time. Adjuvant treatments were also tried. First was lithium, then a series of antipsychotic medications. Thyroid hormone was next, then several other mood stabilizing medications and finally, she returned to trying some of the older antidepressants. Nothing worked.

During this time, the possibility of treatment with electroconvulsive therapy (ECT) was raised. Jane and her family were reluctant to go down this path. As drug treatment after drug treatment failed, their resolve progressively lessened. Anything would be better than the hellish existence Jane was experiencing. Day after day of bleak nothingness. No capacity to laugh, smile, or feel the warmth of the sunshine. No willingness to cuddle the grandkids, to tickle them and walk them through the garden.

Eventually, despite her concerns, she decided to try ECT and checked into a private hospital in an inner suburb of Adelaide. Jane began, as most patients do, with ECT on the right side of her brain. She had a total of nine of these treatments over the course of three weeks. She tolerated the treatment reasonably well but unfortunately experienced no meaningful improvement in the severity of her depression. She was then changed to bilateral ECT: a more potent form of the treatment that is applied to both sides of the brain. Bilateral ECT is the most effective type of ECT but also produces the greatest impact on memory. She had eight of these treatments. They also didn't work. They did, however, produce significant memory impairment. By the eighth treatment, Jane was struggling to remember what happened on treatment days, and in general, life was becoming a bit of a blur. After eight treatments the decision was made to cease the ECT.

This left Jane in a precarious situation. ECT had been described to her as a treatment of last resort and it too had failed. Further medications were offered and explored over the coming months, but nothing produced any substantial benefit. She was sent to a number of different specialists for opinions as to her treatment options. Further ECT was suggested and even more medication trials. Then one day a new psychiatrist suggested something that Jane had not previously heard of. He told her that doctors in Melbourne were experimenting with a new type of treatment for depression: deep brain stimulation (DBS). He explained that DBS was widely used in the treatment of a number of neurological disorders, like Parkinson's disease, and now was being tested as a treatment for depression. Jane and her husband were apprehensive when they first heard about DBS, but with no other treatment options available they agreed to be referred for an assessment.

DBS is a treatment procedure that involves the neurosurgical implantation of very fine wires into the brain, which on one end have very small electrode contacts and on the other end are connected to a pacemaker type device, which is implanted under the skin on the chest. Although DBS is now fairly commonly used for the treatment of Parkinson's disease, the first attempt to implant an electrode in the brain to treat a patient was actually done with the intention to treat depression and anorexia: in an elderly female patient back in 1947. A single electrode was implanted during a neurosurgical procedure, and this functioned for about eight weeks until the electrode wire broke. Whilst working, the system did seem to produce some benefits.

Through the 1960s and 1970s, a number of researchers explored the use of DBS for the treatment of chronic pain although evaluations of its use were far from systematic. In the 1970s and 80s, interest began to grow in the potential use of DBS to treat movement problems such as chronic tremors and Parkinson's disease. At this time, lesional surgery (destroying a small part of the brain) was being used for patients with these disorders, with some success. During one part of the operative procedure, electrical activity from the brain would be recorded prior to the process of destroying a small area of brain tissue. Following the recording of the electrical activity, the implanted wires could be used to electrically stimulate the same area of the brain to test the effects of this stimulation on brain function. In the mid-1970s it was noted that low frequencies of stimulation made tremors worse but stimulation with high frequencies seemed to temporarily improve the clinical profile of patients. From this observation, it was a relatively logical extension to think that electrodes could be used to more permanently stimulate the brain with therapeutic intent. Over the next two decades, researchers progressively evaluated the implantation of electrodes at a series of brain sites involved in movement control, mostly in patients with Parkinson's disease. These techniques have been progressively refined over decades and now DBS is widely used in clinical practice for patients with Parkinson's disease who are suffering despite medication treatment.

The first modern attempt to use DBS in the treatment of a mental health condition occurred in patients with obsessive-compulsive disorder (OCD). In the 1990s OCD was the one remaining mental health condition that was still being treated with lesional surgery. Lesional surgery was the "modern" descendant of the "frontal lobotomy." Lobotomies were widely performed around the world in the in the 1950s and early 1960s, often with terrible outcomes. The procedures were used to try and treat multiple mental health conditions and with limited or no regulatory control in many countries. Their use fortunately waned as medication treatments became more widely available and a public backlash against this form of intervention progressively grew. However, lesional approaches did not die out completely but did become more refined with a focus on placing very small lesions in the brain to interrupt specific connections between different brain regions. OCD was the main remaining condition for which these surgeries continued to be conducted at the time DBS was growing in use.

Given the continued use of a surgical procedure for the treatment of OCD, it is perhaps not surprising that the idea of using DBS came up first for this mental health condition. Throughout the 2000s, DBS began to replace the lesional approach for OCD, with the hope that any ill effects would be reversible (by stopping stimulation), something clearly not possible if a hole had been placed in the brain. DBS seemed to help some patients with their OCD symptoms and over time it was increasingly noticed that when DBS was used in OCD, some patients also experienced significant improvements in mood or even a resolution of depression (patients with OCD frequently will experience substantial episodes of depression as well as their core symptoms of OCD). The latter observation, and our increasing knowledge about the role of specific brain regions in causing depression, paved the way for the first attempts to test DBS in the treatment of depression itself.

About five years after Jane first became depressed, she and her husband came to see me to talk about DBS. We were running a DBS trial at the time, and she seemed a reasonable candidate. Jane was interviewed independently by myself and another psychiatrist, she participated in psychological and neuropsychological assessments and met with the neurosurgeon who would undertake the procedure if she went ahead. Jane remained apprehensive about the procedure but interested in participating, especially motivated by her perception that there were no real other meaningful treatment options still available to her. We told her that DBS was experimental but up to 50% of patients trying the procedure in some trials overseas for depression had received some benefit. There were no guarantees, but for Jane, there were enough reasons to try.

In Victoria, where Jane was to undergo the procedure, DBS if it is used in the treatment of a psychiatric disorder such as depression was defined at the time as a type of "psychosurgery." This meant that its use is highly regulated by the Victorian Mental Health Act and that doctors proposing to perform this procedure were required to apply for approval to the Victorian Psychosurgery review board (since the time Jane underwent the procedure the legislative requirements and adjudicating board have changed). Applying to the review board was a complex process involving a lengthy application that took many weeks to prepare.

### Regulations and DBS

Regulations controlling the use of DBS very dramatically differ around the world. There are places where it, considered as a form of psychosurgery, has been completely made illegal and there are other places where there is little if any formal regulatory control. As we were providing DBS to someone participating in a clinical trial, the approval of this trial also had to be approved by a Human Research and Ethics Committee.

Of note, I am not aware that there is any jurisdiction where the treatment of a patient undergoing DBS for a neurological application such as Parkinson's disease requires any form of regulatory review. This is notable given that patients with Parkinson's disease can have high rates of depression and also can experience significant cognitive impairment that could affect their capacity to consent. Some patients undergoing regulatory review to obtain access to DBS for depression or OCD have described the process as discriminatory, when comparing their experience to those of patients undergoing this treatment for other indications. However, given the ignoble history of the use of forms of psychosurgery in psychiatry, especially lobotomies, is not necessarily surprising that regulatory regimes exist to ensure that surgical treatments are carefully reviewed when being used for psychiatric indications.

Once Jane's application was completed and submitted, a hearing date was set. Jane and her husband came back to Melbourne to attend this hearing. I presented her case to the board outlining why we thought that DBS was a sensible treatment option. I argued that she clearly had severe depression, she had tried all other possible treatments and was able to provide informed consent to the procedure and in fact was doing so. The board, consisting of a lawyer, psychiatrist, neurosurgeon and member of the general public, asked a series of questions to better understand the situation. These questions were asked of Jane, her husband and myself. The questions were at times confronting for Jane: probing her knowledge of the procedure and her ability to understand what was being proposed, even re-evaluating and questioning her diagnosis. The review board needed to satisfy itself that DBS was being considered as a "treatment of last resort" and that Jane was adequately informed about all risks and benefits. It also needed to confirm that she was providing fully informed consent and doing so voluntarily. After what she experienced as a quite grueling process, the board granted permission for the surgery to proceed.

Having undergone a lengthy series of assessments and a rather long and unpleasant review board hearing, Jane's DBS journey was only just beginning. Before she could undergo the surgery, Jane needed to undertake another series of assessments as part of our research procedures to measure her current level of depression and functioning and she had a high resolution magnetic resonance imaging (MRI) scan to provide a detailed picture of her brain, to aid in the surgical process. She was then admitted to the hospital for the procedure.

On the morning of her operation, under injections of only local anesthetic, a stereotaxic frame was attached through her skin to her skull. This is a rather science fiction looking metal ring, a bit like the ones you sometimes see in movies used in people who have a serious neck fracture. This enabled the surgeon to reliably hold in place his instruments and guide the electrodes being implanted to the right place in the brain. She then had yet another brain scan, this time a computerized tomography (CT) scan, and returned to the operating theatre to wait, with the rather cumbersome metal frame still attached to her head. Meanwhile, the MRI and CT scans were "fused" together in a computer. This gives the neurosurgeon the best picture of her brain and an understanding of where the frame is on her head. He can then plan the route that he will take to place the electrodes in her brain. This process is done slowly and carefully trying to visualize in three dimensions the pathway through her brain to the site where the ends of the electrodes were to be placed. Is critical not to pass through an area of the brain containing a concentration of blood vessels as damaging these could lead to a bleed in the brain, a hemorrhage, or stroke.

Once the planning was over, the procedure began. A significant proportion of Jane's scalp was shaved (something she was not happy about afterwards!), incisions were made in the scalp to expose the bone of the skull, and then a type of surgical drill was used to make two holes in the skull, each about the size of a quarter. At all stages of this process, the surgeon repeatedly applied antiseptic lotion to ensure the sterility of the operation site. Jane's surgeon is well known for going somewhat overboard in this process. He even gets in trouble with theatre management for using too much antiseptic, which is pooled all over the floor by the end of the procedure. He also changed his gown and gloves several times during the operation: I suppose you can never be too careful.

Once the holes were put in place, the most critical part of the operation began, the placement of the electrodes. The frame attached to Jane's head was used to support equipment that would guide the electrodes down the path identified on the planning computer. The surgeon had assistants read out numbers from the computer that were then dialed on knobs on the frame. A thin needle was then lowered slowly down through brain tissue, to the target site. When it was close, a machine was hooked up to the back end of the electrode wire that was outside the head. Through this, we listened to the crackling sounds of individual nerve cells firing, detected at the tip of the wire. This gave some indication that we were in the right place.

And then the most surreal step of all began. To set the scene, Jane had not been fully anesthetized but rather treated with local anesthetic and light sedation. She was now required to wake up fully so that she was aware of what was going on inside the operating theatre. She was lying there on the hard operating table with several drips in her arms, a catheter in her bladder, a frame screwed into the bone of her skull and electrodes projecting down into her brain. She had been like this for hours. The electrodes were then turned on and I asked Jane, "How do you feel?"

As a psychiatrist it's something I ask often, and it had never felt quite as absurd a question as it did at that moment. How could anybody under those circumstances feel anything other than terrible? Or even realize that they do? However, strange as it might seem, Jane's sense of how she felt did change. As the electrodes sitting deep in her brain were turned on, she described the dark veil of depression that had been hanging over her for so many years lifting. She felt lighter, more interested in doing something, in doing anything. She wanted to get up, leave the theatre and go outside. She managed to explain this despite the oxygen mask on her face, the surgical drapes covering almost all of her body, especially her head, and all of the incessant noises, beeps and buzzes of the operating theatre. Different electrode contacts were tested, and different intensities of stimulation trialed. Some of these seemed to work but most did not. It was enough information though, to think that the electrodes were being placed in the right part of the brain and that we were onto something.

The operation finished with Jane finally fully asleep: to allow the implantation of a pacemaker type device in Jane's chest, just under her collarbone. Wires were run under the skin from the pacemaker to the top of her scalp and connected to the electrodes. Everything was closed up and she was sent back to the ward to recover.

Perhaps not surprisingly in these days of overcrowded hospitals, within two days of the completion of the operation, suggestions were made that she was ready for discharge. Certainly, she was safe from an operative point of view but she was exhausted and shaken up by the operation and would take quite a number of weeks to get over it. She went home to do this, cared for by her family and friends. She had this strange device in her brain and body, sitting dormant for now.

About four weeks later Jane returned to Melbourne. It was time to turn her stimulator on. There are no clear rules about how to begin DBS stimulation when it is being used in the treatment of depression or really any mental health condition, and there certainly were none when this was being tried on Jane for the first time. At the end of each electrode wire in the brain, there are four separate "contacts." The system can be programmed for the current to flow from any one of these contacts to another or to pass between multiple contacts. The current can also be programmed to flow from one or more of the contacts back to the pacemaker case. Once you have chosen which contacts to use, you next need to work out the frequency of stimulation to be applied (the number of electrical pulses per second), the width of the electrical pulses, and the intensity (voltage or amplitude) of the current. Overall, there are many hundreds of possibilities for the way that stimulation can be applied and considerable variation in how these are chosen. In some research centers, the process is rigid: a fixed stimulation approach is applied for everybody and adjusted infrequently. This does not allow many options to be tested but does provide time to determine whether patients have responded to each stimulation condition that is tested.

We tried a slightly different approach. For the first few days after stimulation was turned on, we spent several hours per day progressively testing a wide range of stimulation settings. Jane would sit in my office; I would program the stimulator to a certain set of conditions and wait five or ten minutes to see what would happen. Stimulation would then be adjusted further. We did this for hours on end and for days at a time. We did this because at the time I thought that if we could find stimulator settings that would produce an optimal temporary improvement in her mood, these could then be left alone for longer-term treatment. This approach certainly works for a condition like Parkinson's disease: stimulation can be adjusted until the patient has the best clinical outcome (can move more readily) and then be left that way for the long-term, only with fine tuning over time. With depression, it is not as clear whether immediate improvements in mood from this type of short-term stimulation will translate to good long-term outcomes, but in the absence of a better approach, this was how we approached the unknown.

For most of the next three days, Jane sat in my office staring at the floor. As I adjusted her stimulation she repeatedly and glumly reported that nothing had changed. Once she got some tingling in her head but that was about it. We both started to get a little bit disappointed: we had not been able to replicate the experience that Jane had in the operating room.

The third day of this process was a Friday. We started late but continued through several hours of the afternoon. About 3 o'clock something rather remarkable happened. Having effectively done little but stare at the floor for two and a half days, Jane suddenly looked up and down my long narrow office to the far wall. "I didn't notice that you had a photo of your children on that wall," she said, as she continued to look around. There was something different in her eyes, in her face. A spark that had not been there before. A brightness I had not previously seen in her. She said that her mood was better, maybe now five, where it had been one of two out of ten before. I fine-tuned the settings a little bit but did not want to change things too much: this was the most promising effect the stimulation had produced since it had been turned on. At about 4 pm we called it a day. Jane was still feeling better. Not dramatically, but noticeably so. She returned from my office in our research center to the small local private hospital where she was staying whilst undergoing the programming. I went home, hopeful but not wanting to get too excited.

Come Monday I was not disappointed. Jane reported that her mood had been even better throughout the weekend and was probably now up to at least a six, or perhaps even a seven, out of ten. She had done some reading, something she had previously enjoyed but had not been able to do since her illness started. She had spoken to people more than she had done in a long time and was just generally more interested in what was going on around her. Most critically, she was really looking forward to going home and spending time with her husband and family. After some consideration, we decided not to progress with further adjustment of her stimulator but allow her to go home and see what would happen over the coming days and weeks.

The outcome of this was also not at all disappointing. In fact, it was better than any of us could have imagined. Within a week or two, Jane reported that her mood had essentially returned to "normal." Her depression was gone. She felt like a new person, or at least certainly like the person she used to be. Her family was delighted: they had their wife and mother back. We all remained apprehensive for some time; we did not know how long this was going to last. However, as days turned to weeks, turned to months, it all seemed more real and substantial. Her mood remained good: there were bad days, but bad days like we all have. Not days of dread and darkness. She fairly rapidly started to reengage with her old life. First, it was seeing family and friends again. Then her scope became broader. She started to explore how she could re-establish an active role in life. She started to do some volunteer work in her primary local school and help actively to care for her grandchildren.

All remained very well for about 18 months. Then one day out of the blue Jane noticed that dreaded feeling again. A heaviness, darkness, a lack of energy and interest. At first, she did not want to believe it was real, that the depression was returning, but slowly it did. Slowly she began to sink lower and lower. Why was this? What was going on? Was the treatment failing as so many treatments had done before? What now? This seemed to be the end of the road. Why had something that worked so well just stopped working?

The answer was simple: her battery was dead.

The battery in Jane's pacemaker-like device had simply run down: the flow of electricity into her brain had dried up and, just as a kid's toy slows down as it runs out of batteries, or the volume of the radio starts to fade, so did she. Her life energy started to slow down and her spark to fade away. This happened quite quickly but fortunately, there is a straightforward solution. She came back to Melbourne and went back into hospital, this time for a quick and simple operation. The device was replaced, and this time with a newer and fancier model. The new unit also had a rechargeable battery. Before, she could leave the thing alone and forget about it but would have to worry that it might not last for long. Now she had a job to do: every few days she would have to sit for an hour or two holding a paddle type device over it to charge up the battery. This was inconvenient but as a result, the unit would last much longer, hopefully up to 15 years.

Once the device was replaced, she came back to the office for it to be turned back on. We restored it to the same settings as previously and waited a few days. Things got better again, but not quite to the same degree. She still felt low, maybe halfway better. So we turned it up. Not much, just an extra trickle of electricity, a few more millivolts. This did the trick. Within days her spark was back again, and life looked rosy once more.

Jane has remained essentially free from depression ever since, except for when she forgets to recharge and her mood starts to slip a bit. At the time of writing, it has been over nine years and counting. She has fully immersed herself back into life. She is participating in community activities and enjoying her growing grandchildren. She has become politically active and speaks publicly about her experiences with depression.

Although Jane's response has been fantastic, almost miraculous, this unfortunately is not the case with all patients who undergo DBS. In our experience, and in clinical trials conducted around the world, some patients have responded to DBS in a really substantial way, like Jane, whilst others have had a much more limited response. Many others, however, do not respond to this treatment. Although it is quite an intimidating process to contemplate, many patients do see the potential for DBS to be a fairly miraculous cure: what could be more scientific and futuristic than stimulating a tiny critical area of the brain to try to fix depression. However, we are certainly not yet at a place where we can be confident where DBS will fit into the future treatment of depression.

The pathway for DBS to progress from being a promising experimental treatment to something that can be used in standard clinical practice is challenging. Despite Jane's wonderful outcome, and others like it, it is possible that we will never be able to complete the type of research needed to prove definitively that it works. Certainly not in a way that would satisfy regulatory authorities whose job it is to scrutinize and approve new treatments before they can be used outside of research.

The problem is this: the standard of proof for a new treatment is a randomized placebo-controlled, double-blind trial. In this context, placebo controlled means you will get either the "real" treatment or a placebo "fake" treatment. The response of patients to the two forms of treatment is compared to see if the "real" treatment is better than the "fake" treatment. This approach works particularly well for new drugs where the placebo is a sugar pill and can be easily disguised. It might be impossible to do the same thing with DBS, however.

To do a double-blind trial with DBS, you have two choices. First, you could pick a fixed set of stimulation settings. That is, the electrodes, frequency, and current strength you want to use. You would then turn the stimulator on at these settings (or not turn it on for the placebo group) and see what happens over some fixed period of time. The alternative is to spend time like we did trying to find the settings that work best, and then either turn the stimulator on using those settings or not.

The first approach is obviously problematic. If there are hundreds or thousands of possible settings, how likely is it that you will pick the right one for enough people? How likely is it that one size will fit all? Seems a bit of a stretch. The problem with option 2 is a little more subtle. When patients undergo the initial testing of stimulation settings, they get a variety of pleasant and unpleasant sensations from the immediate use of the stimulator. These range from physical sensations like tingling or pins and needles in areas of the body, flushing of the face and upper body to sudden changes, for better or worse, in their mood. These tend to be reliably reproducible should the same stimulation settings be re-used.

Therefore, if we find a setting that produces a lift in mood, and choose to use this for treatment, it will be pretty obvious to the patient when the stimulator is turned back on. It will also be obvious when it is not. This makes "double–blinding" of a clinical trial difficult, if not impossible.

### Does Where You Put the Electrodes Matter?

In the early 2000s, two approaches to the use of DBS in depression emerged at the same time, but adopting quite different targets in the brain. One approach grew out of observations that the mood of OCD patients improved when stimulated in a pathway of the brain known as the internal capsule. Multiple groups around the world exploring the use of DBS for OCD and depression conducted small studies implanting patients in the internal capsule or in brain structures close by including brain areas known as the ventral striatum and the nucleus accumbens.

At the same time, a different approach emerged, not based on the observation of therapeutic improvements in other patients, but based upon findings from brain imaging research. In particular, an area of the brain known as the subgenual anterior cingulate had been found to be overactive in a variety of brain imaging studies of patients with depression. It had also been noted that this brain site consistently seemed to become less active when patients successfully responded to treatment: whether this was with medication or ECT. It seemed to be a relatively critical hub in the network of brain areas involved in depression and so became a target for stimulation.

Notably, the early studies at both of these target sites seem to produce similar responses. About half the patients who received treatment had a good or very good response and this seemed to be relatively consistent over time. These two sites then became the targets used in the two multisite industry sponsored trials conducted by Medtronic and St Jude Medical. The failure of these studies has not completely dampened interest in exploring the use of DBS at the sites, and studies continue. However, research efforts have expanded, exploring whether DBS applied at several other brain regions may also be helpful.

Independent researchers, not funded by the companies making the DBS devices (which are quite expensive) conducted many of the first trials of DBS for depression. Most of these studies were what is called open-label. This means that all patients receive active treatment where there is no placebo treatment and no blinding used, just like we did with Jane. The results of these studies have generally been positive, showing benefits of DBS.

However, two large medical device manufacturing companies have attempted the sort of double–blind trials required to get a new treatment approved for use, Medtronic Ltd and St Jude Medical. Medtronic Ltd commenced a trial across multiple hospitals implanting DBS electrodes at a brain site close to where Jane had her electrodes placed. St Jude Medical, chose a different target site but endeavored to do a similar thing. Both trials involved variants of the first approach I described above: some sort of fixed stimulation arrangement. Both trials cost many millions of dollars to set up and run. Both, unfortunately, failed. And failed in a pretty big way. They were both stopped early when an analysis was done of the outcomes part of the way through each trial indicated that they were unlikely to show any beneficial effect of treatment and that continuing was "futile." This outcome could have been because DBS at the brain sites being tested is genuinely not beneficial. However, I believe that it is just as likely that the stimulation method used for the trials (choosing a fixed stimulation intensity, one size fits all) and the time allowed for the treatment to work, was simply not the right way to use DBS. Unfortunately, as described above, there is not necessarily a clearly better option.

Whether or not there is good clinical trial evidence for the effectiveness of DBS, the striking improvement seen in Jane, and the way this has persisted for her, is a very convincing argument that DBS can help some people. The recurrence of her symptoms spontaneously when her battery ran out, something she was not aware of, is also a very good argument that DBS works for her and that her response has not been due to a placebo effect: that she somehow thought herself better. It does leave a more complex question as to how this could be the case. DBS essentially involves the injection of a small consistent electrical current into a very small and well-defined area of the brain. So how can this change the brain processes involved in a disorder like depression?

As we talked about in Chapter 2, for most of the past 40 years, psychiatry has worked with a theory that depression was caused by an abnormality in one or more of the neurochemicals (neurotransmitters) that nerve cells use to communicate with one another. Most commonly, it was believed that depression was caused by a lack of the neurochemical, serotonin. This idea came from the observation that drugs that increased the amount of serotonin in the brain could be effective in the treatment of depression. However, no studies have ever really found evidence for this missing serotonin, or for reduced levels of any of the other neurotransmitters that are affected by antidepressant drugs.

So, what does cause depression then? As we also discussed, brain scanning studies have shown that depression involves changes in activity in multiple areas of the brain. Some areas are too active, while in others the opposite is the case. This research has come about at a time when we are increasingly seeing the brain as a complex organ that operates as a series of interconnected networks. These networks underpin various brain functions. This is a shift away from seeing a simple relationship between one brain area and one function. Depression is increasingly being thought of as a disorder of dysfunction in one or more of these networks. Dysfunction of the network could arise because an illness process affects one or more individual brain regions that make up the network. Alternatively, the network would not function properly if the mechanisms or pathways connecting brain regions were disrupted. For example, if there was an illness affecting the white matter connections between brain regions. That is, the connecting "wires" or pipes of the brain. It is possible that dysfunction in a very small brain region could potentially have profound flow-on effects around a network producing a wide range of symptoms, something seen in depression.

This model also suggests that electrical stimulation in the right brain region to fix a local abnormality could also result in correction of dysfunction around the network. Due to the interconnectedness of the brain, stimulation of a local brain region could also restore normal activity around a network, even if the electrode was not necessarily placed in the area that was primarily responsible for the dysfunction. Presumably, the most potent effects would be achieved if we could identify and stimulate the most critical nodes or junction points in the most relevant networks.

A variant of this idea proposes that brain networks can exist in one of two possible states. Normal network function is maintained in health but a disruption in a region of the network or some substantial input to the network can throw it out so that the network switches into a dysfunctional pattern of activity. According to this theory, depression would be the expression of one or more brain networks switching into this aberrant state of activity. This could occur for a variety of reasons: a stressful event, like the loss of a job or the death of a spouse, could result in the production of high levels of stress hormones that can affect the function of the network. In a vulnerable person, these could disrupt brain activity in just the right way, leading to depression. Someone else might be genetically predisposed to this pattern of activity emerging. Those resilient individuals we see in daily life, those who seem to survive the worst calamities without a hint of depression or anxiety, might just have networks that are hard to shift out of the "normal" way of being. Those individuals, like Jane, with depression that does not respond to all our usual treatments, it might be the opposite. Their brain networks might become stuck in the wrong way of being. Too stuck for the chemical manipulations of antidepressant drugs, the cajoling of psychotherapy or the rebooting of shock therapy to flip them back on track.

This sort of model provides an interesting explanation for the changes that Jane experienced with DBS. Her network was well and truly stuck: nothing could shift it back to the way it should be. DBS in the right place, in the right way, was the key that undid the lock. Once this happened, the brain naturally and quickly reverted to the state it had been in for the decades prior to Jane first becoming unwell. Hopefully as long as that key remains in the lock, the natural condition of her brain, the healthy state, can predominate and she can remain well. So far, so good.

The persistence of benefit seen in some of the studies with DBS to date is a promising feature of the technique. Jane has not had any suggestion of relapse in over nine years of continuous stimulation. Typically, relapse is a major problem with most depression treatments. Patients can relapse despite taking antidepressant drugs. These help reduce relapse, but only to a limited degree. Of the patients who respond really well to ECT, up to one-half will experience a relapse within six months. If DBS is able to maintain wellness long-term, this could have a major impact on the lives of the more severely ill depression sufferers, allowing them to progressively re-establish lives without the threat of relapse hanging over their heads. This stability is likely to be critical for true long-term recovery—the cumulative impact of recurrent episodes of depression is underestimated—repeated episodes disrupt relationships, career trajectories, and progressively diminish self-esteem. Remaining well over a protracted period of time is the only way to reverse these trends. Hopefully, more patients in the future will be able to achieve this with DBS or other treatments with more persistent effects.

Until then, research will go on to better identify the critical networks to target and explore how best to do this. Modern neuroimaging tools, mostly using MRI based techniques, are able to produce a far more sophisticated map of each individual's brain than ever before. They are able to map patterns of brain function, outline in detail the strength and nature of connections between brain regions, and detect subtle changes in blood flow in areas of the brain. Increasing our understanding of normal brain function simultaneously with expanding our knowledge of the processes of dysfunction underlying depression should substantially improve the application of treatments like DBS.

There is also likely to be a significant improvement in DBS technologies. Current approaches involve the fixed application of electricity through a limited number of four electrode contacts. Research is already underway to develop more sophisticated systems with substantially enhanced numbers of contacts to allow more fine tuning of electrical stimulation.

Finally, it will also be interesting to see how "closed loop" technologies can be applied to the treatment of depression with DBS. Closed loop methods involve the simultaneous recording of electrical activity from neurons in the brain and provision of electrical stimulation. The type of stimulation is determined by the pattern of electrical activity detected. This type of approach is already being applied to the treatment of epilepsy. The closed loop system monitors for electrical activity suggesting the emergence of a seizure, which is then interrupted by an electrical stimulus. One could imagine the development of a system whereby the electrical signal of emerging depressive thoughts could be detected and directly interrupted through DBS to prevent the development of a depressive episode. How ever they develop, the future for these treatment approaches will be interesting to watch.

# 10

# KETAMINE: SHOULD WE BELIEVE THE HYPE?

THE DEVELOPMENT OF ketamine as an antidepressant strategy has been one of the most exciting, overhyped, and concerning innovations in the management of depression in recent years, all at the same time. Tom Insel, former director of the National Institute for Mental Health, has been repeatedly quoted from a 2014 blog as having said ketamine "*might be the most important breakthrough in antidepressant treatment in decades.*"* If ketamine turns out to be a rapidly effective treatment for patients struggling with depression, and can be safely and efficiently supplied to patients, this might just be the case. But there are "*ifs*" there, just as there was a commonly ignored "*might*" in the statement by Tom Insel.

There is good reason for optimism here. Ketamine appears to have considerable potential. In some cases, it appears to lift patients from severe depression in a rapid manner not seen with any other therapeutic options, including ECT. However, the data to date supporting ketamine remains limited. We have highly promising data from short term trials of intravenous administration and a somewhat controversial and limited data set that somehow managed to result in clinical approval for an intranasal version of ketamine in the United States. However, we lack long-term data, especially on safety, and psychiatry has a history of getting rather excited about new treatments before we really know enough about them.

* https://www.nimh.nih.gov/about/directors/thomas-insel/blog/2014/ketamine.shtml

However, it is within this context that clinical services have sprung up like mushrooms, all over the place. Even before the approval of intranasal ketamine, clinics providing intravenous ketamine infusions were setting up around the US and in other places throughout the world. These are often not backwards in promoting the potential of this therapy. "Get your life back," "Reset your brain, reset your life." "In just 72 hours you can get your life back," are all quotes taken from clinic websites I found in a two-minute Google search. Some are run by psychiatrists, some by anesthetists, and some by nurse practitioners or nurse anesthetists. None of these alone has the breadth of skills to manage patients with severe treatment resistant depression and the intravenous administration of a potent drug. Many services do not seem to provide treatment backed by the sort of multi-disciplinary team that you would ideally want to oversee a program like this.

Ketamine treatment is complicated, and there are lots of red flags to suggest patients should tread warily in this area. But what is it? What does it do and what is the evidence supporting all this hype?

Ketamine is a drug that was actually developed a long time ago: first in 1962 by chemists in the Park Davis pharmaceutical company who were attempting to develop new anesthetic agents based upon the drug phencyclidine (PCP). PCP had profound anesthetics effects but had been found to be unsuitable, not least of all because it could induce prolonged excitation after anesthesia and severe disturbing psychotic reactions. It had an excellent profile regarding its effects during anesthesia on the heart and lungs, however, motivating the search for similar but more suitable drugs.

Ketamine was a product of this search. Chemically, it combines a ketone molecule and an amine so was perhaps not so creatively named from these. It was first tested as an anesthetic in Michigan in 1964, and administered to prisoners in the Jackson State prison. Unusual effects of ketamine were noticeable in its very first uses. One in three subjects reported strange experiences, such as feeling like one was floating in outer space. These were described as "dissociative," referring to the idea that subjects would feel disconnected from their experiences, and ketamine later became known as a "dissociative anesthetic."

The use of ketamine was approved by the FDA in the US in 1970 and following this, it was used widely as a battlefield anesthetic during the Vietnam war. As ketamine does not suppress breathing or blood pressure, in general use as an anesthetic and sedative, it was seen to be safer than many other alternative medications, especially in emergency situations that are common in war. It particularly became a popular drug for use in children: either as an anesthetic agent or as a sedative during procedures in emergency departments where sedation might be required during the performance of painful procedures such as resetting of a fracture. It is especially useful under these circumstances as it can be administered as an intramuscular injection when setting up an intravenous infusion is problematic. However, in adult patients as a standalone anesthetic, it suffered from some of the problems that derailed the use of PCP. Patients could wake up with quite disturbing experiences: hallucinations and over excitement were a real issue and its use waned as better tolerated anesthetic drugs like propofol were developed.

Illicit use of ketamine did not take long to emerge. As early as 1971, one year after its official approval for human use, there were reports of its use to produce visual hallucinations and altered sensory experiences, not too dissimilar from the effects of LSD,* and its spread was probably propagated by its common use in Vietnam. In the late 1970s its illicit use was further popularized in books such as *Journeys into a Bright World* by Marcia Moore, a well-known author of new age books, and Howard Alltounian, an anesthetist she met at one of her workshops. The two were married soon after two ketamine "journeys" together and published a book describing their experiences arising from repeated uses of the drug. However, Moore, the self-proclaimed "priestess of the Goddess Ketamine," froze to death on a winters night in 1979 having injected ketamine in a forest, determined as she had told friend, fellow ketamine explorer, and author John Lilly, that she would "ride this comet through to the end."

Illicit use of ketamine was predominately concentrated in the new age community but by the mid-1980s its use grew significantly as part

* https://pubmed.ncbi.nlm.nih.gov/5548039/

of dance club culture. It was often substituted for MDMA (ecstasy) and gained a bad reputation as its effects, especially orally, were often much less pleasant. Ketamine became a controlled substance in the US in 1999 and in Victoria, Australia in the same year. Its illicit use has waxed and waned over the years, never really going away, and its use in well to do young financial professionals has gained some recent notoriety through the UK TV series, *Industry*.

In medical practice, as well as its use as a sedative or anesthetic agent, there were increasing reports from the late 1990s onward that ketamine could be used in the treatment of cancer and non-cancer related chronic pain. Infusions of intravenous ketamine, in particular, became relatively commonly utilized in patients with persistent chronic pain syndromes such as fibromyalgia, complex regional pain syndrome, and phantom limb pain. This use of ketamine has persisted to the current day, with anesthetists interested in the management of chronic pain, commonly providing this as a clinical service. It is this expertise that appears, in places, to have led the same professionals to offer intravenous infusions for the treatment of depression, despite a lack of training in the management of mental health conditions.

That is all well and good but what about using ketamine for depression? Why was this even proposed? Well, ketamine acts as a blocker of the N-methyl-D-aspartate (NMDA) receptor for the neurotransmitter glutamate. Glutamate is actually by far the most common neurotransmitter (neurochemical) in the human brain. It is the chemical that is involved in most "excitatory" neurotransmission in the brain: in other words, when one nerve cell sends a signal to stimulate (make fire) a second nerve cell, chances are it is using glutamate to do this. However, this has little to do with the so-called NMDA receptor. When glutamate is involved in this excitatory activity, it acts at other receptors (not the NMDA one) at the same time, all with equally silly names. However, when glutamate binds to these other receptors, it will also attach to some NMDA receptors which are found on the same nerve cells. Activation of the NMDA receptor, especially when nerve cells are repeatedly stimulated, tends to be involved in self-regulatory processes: tuning up or tuning down the likelihood that these nerve cells will fire when stimulated in the future. It is like activation of the NMDA receptor is part of a process of cell "memory": remembering that the cell has been repeatedly stimulated, and then triggering some action in response to this.

In the mid-1990s, there was an emerging theoretical idea that changes in the NMDA receptor might be involved in the cause of depression. Early animal studies suggested that drugs that could block the action of glutamate at the NMDA receptor might have antidepressant activity and it was noted that other antidepressant drugs also might affect this particular receptor. Therefore, researchers were interested in exploring whether drugs used to specifically target the NMDA receptor system could have antidepressant effects in human patients.

So they looked around for options, and as it turns out, Ketamine just happens to be an effective blocker of the NMDA receptor and one that by the late 1990s was widely available for researchers to test.

The first study to do this was published by researchers at Yale University in the year 2000.* Nine patients with depression participated in a study which involved them receiving two intravenous infusions each for 40 minutes. On one day, they received an infusion of ketamine and on the second day, they received just a saltwater infusion. They were not told whether they received the active drug or not. The dose of ketamine used was not high enough to anesthetize the patients but did produce significant subjective symptoms including effects on thinking and mood during the time of the infusion, making "blinding" of the patients in this research somewhat problematic. In other words, they probably knew when they received the ketamine and when they did not.

Most importantly, active ketamine treatment was associated with a fairly dramatic short-term improvement in depression. Four of the eight patients experienced a reduction in depression scores sufficient enough to be considered clinical response and the same improvement was seen in only one patient following the placebo infusion. Most impressively, and unlike anything seen in other lines of depression therapy research,

* Berman RM, Cappiello A, Anand A, Oren DA, Heninger GR, Charney DS, Krystal JH. Antidepressant effects of ketamine in depressed patients. Biol Psychiatry. 2000 Feb 15;47(4):351-4. doi: 10.1016/s0006-3223(99)00230-9.

improvement was seen within 24 hours of the infusion and was still present three days later. However, the patient's depression had returned to the baseline level of severity one week later.

Since the publication of this study, understandably there has been rapid growth in interest in the potential application of ketamine as a novel antidepressant. Several similar studies, applying single intravenous doses, have found similar effects: ketamine appears capable of producing a rapid onset of powerful antidepressant effects even in patients who have struggled to respond to other therapies. The benefits are seen in patients with major depression, as well as for patients in the depressive phase of bipolar affective disorder, and can be associated with a rapid reduction in suicidal ideation. However, following a single treatment, these antidepressant effects are relatively short lived. These studies have also been criticized as they are not seen to be adequately "controlled." In other words, the patients could be getting better due to strong placebo effects. This appears possible as most patients receiving ketamine will experience subtle, or in some cases dramatic, effects on their thinking, including the dissociation mentioned before. Patients receiving a saltwater infusion as a placebo will not have these effects and as such, patients in these studies are likely to be aware when they are having the real thing.

There is an additional critical issue: the short-term nature of the effects seen. Clearly, a more important question than whether ketamine can work in the short-term is whether there are ways of using it that can be applied to achieve meaningful long-term clinical benefits. There have been attempts to do this although there remain very few published studies of the effects of repeated infusions of intravenous ketamine (despite the overwhelming claims of some of the clinics offering this service). In one example, a group of researchers gave 18 patients with severe depression either electroconvulsive therapy or three infusions of ketamine with a two day break between treatments. Antidepressant effects came on quickly with the ketamine treatment, only after one treatment, faster than benefits from ECT, and were of a similar magnitude at the end of the week of therapy. This one week of treatment, however, was still relatively short-term. Not all studies have demonstrated that repeated administrations of intravenous ketamine are effective in relieving depression. In a recent study from the Massachusetts General Hospital in Boston, 26 patients with severe depression received either six ketamine infusions or placebo infusions over three weeks.* This study failed to show any difference between active ketamine and placebo despite using the standard dose that has been utilized in most previous studies.

At this stage, the only logical conclusion from this body of research is that the jury is still out: it remains unclear whether repeated intravenous infusions of ketamine really work. There are many outstanding and critical questions including 1) can repeated infusions be used to induce complete remission of depression (and if so, how many are required and how frequently should these be administered), 2) can regular infusions of ketamine then be used to prevent the return of the illness (and again, if so, how often do these need to be), 3) and, is this actually safe? Are there adverse effects that emerge with ongoing treatment? Will repeated use in a medical setting lead to problems with addiction and dependence like those that led Marcia Moore into that frozen forest back in 1979?

Unfortunately, we are going to have to wait until these questions are adequately answered with decent research, and in the meantime, given the expanding clinical use, hope that there are not significant adverse consequences that will accumulate over time. Given the horrendous consequences of the ongoing opioid epidemic, also something that arose from therapeutic good intentions, let's hope unrestricted use of intravenous ketamine is not going to germinate similar challenges for the future.

Are there options other than having to inflict repeated injections of ketamine on patients? Well, given the limitations of intravenous ketamine administration, it is not surprising that attempts have been made to try and develop other ways of providing this therapy. What about taking it in oral (tablet or liquid) form? This is possible but most of the ketamine taken orally is metabolized rapidly as it passes through the liver

* Ionescu DF, Bentley KH, Eikermann M, et al. Repeat-dose keta-mine augmentation for treatment-resistant depression with chronic suicidal ideation: a randomized, double blind, placebo-controlled trial. J Affect Disord.2019;243:516–524. doi:10.1016/j.jad.2018.09.037

before being distributed to the rest of the body. In the liver, ketamine is mostly broken down into a different compound, norketamine. However, this may have some antidepressant activity itself and oral administration would be much, much better than intravenous.

There have been a number of studies on various forms of oral ketamine and this type of formulation continues to be the focus of commercial drug development. For example, in 2018 a group of Iranian researchers published the results of a trial where 90 patients were given either oral ketamine (50mg/day) plus the antidepressant, sertraline, or placebo plus sertraline, all daily for six weeks. Patients receiving the ketamine responded faster, had a greater overall response rate, and had less depression at weeks 2, 4, and 6. The oral ketamine was tolerated very well, without dissociative or other serious symptoms. Unfortunately, this paper tells us nothing about what happened to the patients after the 6 weeks of treatment. At the time of writing, a substantial study was underway, sponsored by the New Zealand based company, Douglas Pharmaceuticals, evaluating the use of an extended release oral ketamine formulation.

The other form of ketamine administration which has attracted considerable, and successful, commercial development, has been intranasal administration. In 2019, Janssen pharmaceutical company announced that the FDA in the US had approved the clinical use of "esketamine" nasal spray for patients with treatment resistant depression, sold under the trade name of *Spravato*: I will discuss a little later why this was *es*ketamine and what this means.

This approval was based on two clinical studies: in the first, intranasal esketamine commenced at the same time as a new oral antidepressant produced a greater improvement in depression than if patients only received an intranasal placebo plus the new medication over four weeks (with treatment three times per week). This was followed by a second, longer term study, where patients who achieved remission on intranasal esketamine demonstrated a lower long-term relapse rate than patients who received placebo medication. FDA approval of esketamine in the US has resulted in clinical marketing of the drug but under circumstances where it can only be administered in a "certified facility" and where patients must be observed and monitored for at least two hours after taking the drug each time.

The approval process of esketamine has not been without controversy and the company has not been successful with subsequent applications in some other countries. There have been several issues. First was an issue with the process of approval itself. In an earlier chapter, I described how the FDA has historically required two positive trials of a medication as a demonstration of efficacy prior to approval. However, that standard was not maintained in the approval process of esketamine. As noted above, the approval was based upon only one study demonstrating the efficacy of the medication and this was in short-term use, supported by the longer-term relapse prevention data. Two other studies of the acute use of esketamine were conducted but actually failed to show benefits of the drug above and beyond that seen with placebo medication.*

There were also criticisms of the actual trial data itself. In the single positive acute treatment study, esketamine only improved depression by four points (on the 60 point MADRS scale) greater than placebo, a relatively weak effect. The challenge with showing esketamine was better than placebo was exacerbated by about half of the patients receiving placebo improving to a point where they were considered treatment responders. Overall, 81% of the response to esketamine was considered to have also been seen with placebo treatment.** High placebo response rates are a major problem with all antidepressant medication studies. It was likely that responses were especially high in the placebo group in this trial because patients did not just receive a placebo. Remember, they were also commenced on a new antidepressant medication at the same time that they commenced esketamine. This may not have been much of a concern if the patients were very treatment resistant and had failed lots of medication trials, as the likelihood of improving with the antidepressant medication would be low. However, the patients in this

---

\* https://www.thelancet.com/journals/lanpsy/article/PIIS2215-0366(19)30292-5/fulltext
\*\* https://www.thelancet.com/journals/lanpsy/article/PIIS2215-0366(19)30394-3/fulltext

trial were not all that resistant to antidepressant medication. Therefore, it is not at all surprising that a group of the patients on placebo just got better with the antidepressant pills alone, a real problem with the actual trial design itself.

You might be a little surprised that the study was done in patients not considered all that treatment resistant, especially as the potential benefits of ketamine in really difficult to treat patients is often proposed as its great advantage. However, in this study, patients only had to have failed two medications, and these did not even have to be of differing medication types. In fact, almost a quarter of the patients in the trial had only failed two medications of one single drug type. There were also significant concerns about whether subjects really were adequately unaware of which treatment they were on. As already discussed, ketamine produces quite distinct effects, and it is likely that a substantial proportion of patients in the study would have been aware of whether they were receiving the active drug or the placebo.

One other feature of this study has also gathered considerable attention. During the main efficacy study of 227 patients, there were six deaths, including three by suicide. Suicide is an unfortunate consequence of severe depression, but given that patients who had significant suicidal ideation or actions in the 12 months prior to the study were actually excluded from participation, these rates do seem unusually high. As a realistic comparator, no deaths by suicide were seen in the roughly 700 patients who participated in the main trials of TMS therapy in depression. These patients are likely to have relatively similar characteristics. Contradicting the results of previous research with intravenous ketamine, in this study esketamine did not show a benefit greater than placebo in actually reducing suicidal ideation. Professor Alan Schatzberg from Stanford University recently speculated that the use of ketamine might be associated with a serious withdrawal reaction, especially given that some research has suggested that ketamine interacts with opioid receptors in the brain: the site of action of drugs such as heroin and morphine.* Notably, the deaths by suicide occurred four, twelve and

* https://ajp.psychiatryonline.org/doi/10.1176/appi.ajp.2019.19040423

twenty days *after* the patient's last dose of esketamine. None occurred during treatment or during or after cessation of placebo. This specific timing supports the idea that these effects could be withdrawal related: that patients experience suicidal thoughts as part of some form of withdrawal reaction from the drug.

A final disappointing aspect of the esketamine studies is that they really failed to demonstrate a rapid onset of the antidepressant effects of esketamine, something that has really attracted a lot of attention to this treatment approach. In one of the Janssen studies, only 10% of patients who received ketamine experienced a rapid clinical response and in most of the studies, there was no meaningful early difference between active drug and placebo.*

Despite these concerns, Janssen has had considerable success with its rollout of esketamine treatment and reported more than 850 certified treatment centers around the US by late 2019.** This has been a considerably politicized process. In mid-2019 the US Department of Veterans Affairs had to make a decision as to whether esketamine would be included on the list of drugs that could be used within the veterans' health care system. In the lead up to the decision-making process, President Donald Trump told Veterans Affairs secretary Robert Wilkie that he believed that the treatment could result in an "incredible drop" in veterans' suicide rates and offered to personally help negotiate pricing with Janssen.

Trump was quoted as saying, "You have people calling for help and if those people had that (esketamine), I'm hearing like instantaneously they're in better shape."***

Despite this high level intervention, the clinical panel within the Department of Veterans Affairs did not add esketamine to the general

---

* https://www.thelancet.com/journals/lanpsy/article/PIIS2215-0366(19)30394-3/fulltext
** https://www.fiercepharma.com/pharma/j-j-scores-spravato-trial-win-high-risk-depression-will-doctors-and-payers-buy
*** https://www.bloomberg.com/news/articles/2019-06-12/trump-offers-to-negotiate-price-of-j-j-anti-depressant-for-va

formulary but instead established a process requiring prior authorization and strict administration requirements.

Related to this, there have been concerns about the pricing of *Spravato*. The Boston-based Institute for Clinical and Economic Review, which provides an independent appraisal of the cost benefits of treatments, concluded in mid-2019 that *Spravato* was being marketed at a cost that was substantially in excess of a price at which it would be considered cost-effective: at its marketed price of $32,400 per year it was "low value for money."*

These concerns about efficacy and the clinical trials exploring the effects of both intravenous and intranasal forms of ketamine sit in contrast to the multitude of first-hand stories from patients who report dramatic benefits of the drug. There are numerous media stories describing excellent ketamine related outcomes achieved by individual patients and countless testimonials fill the websites of commercial clinics offering the therapy.

However, what is it actually like to undertake this form of treatment? Well the experience will certainly differ with the mode of administration: having an intravenous drip put in place is more complicated than using a nasal spray (although the drip does guarantee a more consistent dose as people do not always coordinate intranasal administration well). The side effects are likely to be similar, but what are these?

First, as already described, there are the odd experiences and emotions one may feel post dosing. A patient's mood can go quickly up, but the opposite effects are sometimes seen. Hallucinations may occur: these are the presence of false perceptions that you may see, hear or even feel. Dissociation is more common than full blown hallucinations. During dissociation, people can experience being meaningfully disconnected from one's thoughts, feelings, or sense of identity. They can feel mildly odd or much more profoundly disturbed, they can really "trip out." Dissociation was reported in over 30% of patients taking esketamine in one study.** Other common side effects reported in clinical trials include

---

* https://icer-review.org/announcements/trd_final_report/
** https://adaa.org/sites/default/files/Canuso-AJP-2018.pdf

sedation (remember this is an anesthetic drug), dizziness, headache, anxiety, nausea, and vomiting. There are also several risks of ketamine identified in people who abuse the drug. These include an inflammation of the bladder and liver. It remains unclear how much of a problem these will be with more common clinical use of the drug but some people having repeatedly abused ketamine have developed major problems with their bladder, the so called *K Bladder*, even requiring surgical removal in some cases.

The dissociation described is not a trivial side-effect of ketamine, certainly one that can cause both immediate and ongoing distress to patients and was presumably one of the motivating factors in the FDA requiring a significant period of observation of a patient after esketamine dosing. To illustrate this, I would like to tell you a little bit about a patient called Dane who I saw several years ago. Dane was participating in a clinical trial of a form of ketamine, although in this case, not esketamine. Dane was in his early 30s and had a long and troublesome history of treatment resistant depression that had persisted for over eight years. During that time he had tried an extensive range of standard antidepressants, a series of atypical antipsychotic agents, and several mood stabilizers including lithium. He had not been willing to try electroconvulsive therapy at this stage of his illness but had had an unsuccessful course of high-frequency left-sided TMS. He had approached our research center when he had heard about the ketamine study that we were undertaking having read previously about its potential benefits on the Internet. He was extremely keen to participate in the study and after the appropriate screening, was consented and enrolled in the trial.

Dane's first couple doses of ketamine went relatively smoothly. However, he reported no real change in his mood during these treatment sessions. However, things changed dramatically when he received treatment at a higher dose, as he was scheduled to do in the protocol given his non-response to treatment up until that time. About 30 minutes after receiving this third dose he became increasingly distressed and confused. He described not really understanding what was going on around him and started to act in an unpredictable and disorganized fashion. Within another five minutes or so he had gotten down onto the floor and was crawling around on his hands and knees not really responding in an understandable manner to the staff members who were trying to take care of him or able to explain what he was doing. This went on for some time before he gradually settled down, was able to be reassured, and slowly over the course of an hour or so his mental state returned to normal.

This was clearly very distressing for him although his memories of what he underwent were quite patchy afterwards. It was probably a good thing that he did not really remember exactly what he was doing during this time as I suspect that this would have been even more disturbing.

Of note, the occurrence of this event did not really diminish Dane's interest and motivation in continuing with ketamine treatment. Ketamine treatment does appear to be of particular attraction to a certain group of patients. Most patients undergoing this treatment in my experience have had it recommended by a psychiatrist as would happen with any other form of intervention. However, there are a smaller, but significant, group of patients who—having read about ketamine, usually on the Internet—are highly driven to access it as a treatment and at times will often push extremely hard to achieve access. There is clearly going to be some degree of overlap between these patients and those who have experienced the use of ketamine as a drug of abuse previously and teasing these issues out I think will prove to be a challenge for those prescribing ketamine in the future.

As I was discussing the clinical evidence above, I very much glossed over the difference between ketamine and esketamine, focusing on the fact that the latter has been developed as a drug administered through an intranasal spray. However, esketamine and ketamine are not exactly the same thing. Ketamine is a specific type of chemical that is made up of two "enantiomers." Enantiomers are a pair of molecules that are identical mirror images of one another, just as one of your hands is the mirror image of the other. They are the same but not the same. A number of different drugs are made up of two enantiomers and in some cases, the enantiomers have been separated to allow one of these to be marketed as a separate drug. For example, the antidepressant citalopram is made up of two enantiomers and one of these was isolated and produced as a separate antidepressant, escitalopram, around the time that the original drug was coming out of patent protection.

Ketamine is effectively made up of two enantiomers which are referred to as the S-ketamine and R-ketamine molecules. Esketamine is effectively the S-ketamine component of the full mix of S and R ketamine. Therefore, it is not necessarily possible to directly compare the results of studies using more traditional intravenous R+S ketamine to the intranasal esketamine developed by Janssen. Interestingly, there have been studies that would have suggested that using R-ketamine may have been a more effective strategy than S-ketamine alone. A very early study conducted in the 1990s indicated that S-ketamine was associated with significant psychiatric side effects including dissociation and hallucinations but these same adverse effects were not produced with R-ketamine. More recent studies have suggested that R+S ketamine may have longer acting therapeutic action compared to S-ketamine alone. A recent small study in Brazil tested the effects of R-ketamine with promising results.* A persistence in antidepressant effects was seen after a single infusion for up to 7 days in some patients. This does seem to be longer than what we might otherwise expect but this is very early research.

Unfortunately, at this stage, the best we can say about this topic is that we really don't know what is likely to prove to be the best form of ketamine, both in terms of the molecule itself and the form of delivery. There is clearly a substantial need for meaningful ongoing research, and, especially given the increasing clinical use of forms of ketamine, that this research is done quickly and comprehensively. It is regrettably true, however, that the increasing clinical availability of ketamine makes this much more problematic. When treatment is available clinically, it is much more difficult to engage patients in important research trials than before. If they can access it freely, why participate in a clinical trial?

And ketamine is certainly increasingly clinically available, especially in the US. In fact, the limited clinical and research evidence has really failed to slow down the dramatic escalation in clinical services providing access to ketamine therapy. Even prior to the FDA's approval of *Spravato*,

* https://pubmed.ncbi.nlm.nih.gov/32078034/

the provision of ketamine in relatively unregulated clinics was dramatically expanding. A 2018 investigation by the website STAT, which sits within the Scientific American family, found some really worrying characteristics of clinics that have popped up offering intravenous ketamine infusions throughout the US.*

First, there seems to be a considerable degree of variability in the clinical oversight within these services. Some appear to have no meaningful medical psychiatric supervision and might just be run by an anesthetically trained doctor or even a nurse practitioner. An anesthetist may be perfectly trained to supervise the actual mechanics of a ketamine infusion but will not have the expertise to adequately assess and screen patients or manage the potential adverse behavioral results of therapy. This failing appears to be exacerbated by a significant disconnect between the therapy offered by many of these clinics and the day-to-day mental health management of patients.

Treatment within these clinics is also expensive, running at up to $1000 per infusion often with six infusions provided on a regular basis plus additional top-ups as required. STAT also outlined how clearly ketamine therapy is overhyped by many of these services, often with misleading quotes on websites and in promotional materials. Treatment is often widely promoted through social media and intake and screening processes can be scanty. This is likely to be a major problem if clinics are attracting drug seeking patients.

The development of these sorts of clinical programs is not a uniquely a US phenomenon. A series of clinics in Australia were shut down in 2015 following an investigation by health authorities and ABC media which identified some rather dubious practices. Ketamine was provided with minimal medical oversight and some patients were sent home with syringes for self-administration, a recipe for drug diversion into illicit use.

In this context, it is at least reassuring that the FDA in the US has only allowed *Spravato* to be administered through certified clinics as part

---

* https://www.scientificamerican.com/article/is-the-ketamine-boom-getting-out-of-hand/

of a Risk Evaluation and Mitigation Strategy mandated by the FDA. This may seem to be too restrictive to some but given the degree to which there is potential for inappropriate use of ketamine, it seems to be a sensible and well justified precaution.

So, what can we say, at this stage about the clinical utility of ketamine and when should it be considered in the management of depression? If it is used, in what patients is it most likely to be suitable, and how should it be administered? In some places, this is not an issue right now as ketamine in any form is not yet widely available clinically although this is now very much an issue in the US.

My take is that ketamine does have a role but at this stage, the uncertainty around its long-term safety leaves this as a fairly limited one. There is, as has been repeatedly the focus in this book, a pressing need for new and improved therapeutics for patients who don't respond to initial antidepressant medications. Therefore, it is critical to be open to new interventions. However, the overall evidence base for the efficacy of ketamine is quite limited and there are substantial concerns about the possibility of long-term side effects, emergent risks around suicidality, and dependence.

The best way to balance these issues is with careful and thorough clinical procedures. Patients should receive a thorough psychiatric assessment prior to engaging in ketamine therapy to balance this option with the other available interventions, things such as TMS therapy and ECT. Risk factors for substance dependence should be evaluated as well as those associated with emergent suicidal ideation. The support available to the individual, their capacity to recognize clinical deterioration, and access these supports should be carefully considered.

The second and most critical element is the provision of really thorough information prior to patient consent. Patients should be informed about the potential benefits of ketamine but also the limitations of the evidence supporting its use, the known side effects, and the uncertainty about long-term safety. Patients really need to be provided with information about the other therapeutic options and how ketamine fits into the overall picture.

I am afraid the proliferation of ketamine only clinics, especially those without meaningful psychiatric involvement, makes the universal achievement of these standards somewhat unlikely. Under these circumstances, my advice to patients is to carefully "shop around." Ask lots of questions, read widely, and do not hesitate to get second or third opinions if you are unsatisfied. If something is being sold as "too good to be true," this is likely to be the case: ketamine may change your life but just be careful!

| SIDE EFFECTS OF KETAMINE | | |
|---|---|---|
| **Psychiatric** | Low mood, hallucinations, dissociation | These are common and dose-related |
| **Visual** | Blurred vision or seeing double | |
| **Gastrointestinal** | Nausea and vomiting | Seen in about one in five patients in some studies |
| **Other brain related** | Headache | |
| **Urinary** | Bladder inflammation (cystitis) | Seen in individuals who abuse ketamine, rates and clear in therapeutic use. |
| **Liver** | Liver inflammation | Some evidence that this also occurs in individuals who abuse ketamine |

# 11

# THE PROMISE OF PSYCHEDELIC-ASSISTED PSYCHOTHERAPY

ALTHOUGH KETAMINE ACHIEVED a degree of community recognition and awareness as a drug of illicit use in the 1970s and 1980s, its popularity and notoriety have always been relatively insignificant compared to the uses of another group of drugs which are enjoying a renaissance as potential therapies for mental health conditions, including depression: the psychedelics. Psychedelic drugs are substances that produce mind altering, especially mind "expanding," effects. They may change our perception, how we see and take in the world around us, heighten awareness and the flow and content of thoughts. The modern rediscovery of the use of psychedelic drugs in psychiatry involves their use to enhance or facilitate a specific psychotherapeutic process, called psychedelic-assisted psychotherapy or psychedelic therapy.

There are quite a number of well known, and less well known, psychedelic drugs but a much smaller range of these are being meaningfully developed therapeutically. LSD (lysergic acid diethylamide) is often considered the classical or archetypal psychedelic. However, as the product of a chemical laboratory—synthesized in the 1940s by the Swiss company Sandoz—its use evolved much more recently than other naturally derived compounds which in some cases have been used for thousands of years. The potential for LSD to be used as a therapeutic agent in mental health disorders was recognized as far back as the 1940s. In the 20 years after its first synthesis, experiments were done using LSD in healthy individuals as well as patients with various mental health conditions. It became clear through this experimental use, and later more widespread illicit use, that LSD can produce quite profound changes in perception, including visual and auditory hallucinations: seeing and hearing things that are not there. Experiments investigating the use of LSD, especially in the US, formally ceased in 1968 when its possession and use were curtailed by drug control regulations.

## Hofmann and the Discovery of LSD

Five years after Albert Hofmann first synthesized LSD in the laboratories at Sandoz, he decided to conduct a series of experiments to investigate its properties. He later recounted that on the day of these experiments he described feeling like he was "being affected by a remarkable restlessness, combined with a slight dizziness. At home I lay down and sank into a not unpleasant, intoxicated-like condition characterized by an extremely stimulated imagination." Thinking this was an effect of the drug, three days later he took 250 micrograms of the drug to confirm the effect. Not feeling well, and without any other mode of transport, Hofmann embarked on what has become a fairly famous bicycle ride home.

He felt dizzy, had a changed sense of vision and perceived that he was barely moving, although others reported him riding fast. At home things got worse. He described "powerful motor disturbances, alternating with paralysis...a feeling of suffocation; confusion alternating with clear recognition of my situation, in which I felt outside myself as a neutral observer as I half-crazily cried or muttered indistinctly." This eventually faded and he realized this was an extraordinary substance. Over the next year Hoffman took small doses, 20-30 micrograms, at least four times with mixed effects. In 1944, Werner Stoll, a psychiatrist and son of Hoffman's boss took a dose of 60 micrograms, and had what was the first truly psychedelic (and pleasant) trip resulting from the use of LSD.

In contrast to LSD, DMT (N,N-Dimethyltryptamine) is a naturally derived substance, the main ingredient in ayahuasca. Taken alone, DMT produces an intense but short lived psychedelic effect, often as short at five or ten minutes when inhaled. In ayahuasca, DMT is typically combined with a second compound which acts to substantially delay its metabolism significantly enhancing the duration of the psychedelic effects produced. There is clear evidence that ayahuasca has been used in South America for at least 1000 years for ritualistic and healing purposes. In keeping with other psychedelic substances, the effects induced by ayahuasca are described as being highly dependent on the user's expectations as well as the environment in which the drug is taken. Euphoria, altered sensations, and mystical experiences are widely reported but use can also be associated with the induction of psychotic episodes, especially in individuals with a background of mood or substantial mental health problems.

Psilocybin is another naturally derived psychedelic and one that is now being actively developed for therapeutic use. Psilocybin is produced in over 200 species of mushrooms and is the active ingredient in "magic mushrooms." Psilocybin itself does not produce psychedelic effects but is converted in the body to psilocin which does. Its effects include elevated mood, hallucinations, altered perception and sense of time, and profound spiritual experiences. Its use, like that of DMT, is also ancient and is believed to date back before recorded history, as evidenced by rock paintings and murals found in Spain and Algeria. Psilocybin, was first chemically isolated in Sandoz in 1959, the pharmaceutical company that invented LSD, by the chemist Albert Hofmann. It continues to be used illicitly in its natural form and is being synthesized by a number of pharmaceutical companies to supply an increasing market in investigational therapeutic trials.

A second "reinvented" drug being actively tested for therapeutic benefits is not traditionally considered a classical psychedelic drug. 3,4- methylenedioxymethamphetamine (MDMA or ecstasy) is often called an "enactogen" or "empathogen" due to its capacity to increase emotional connection, a sense of oneness and emotional openness. This usually comes without the same degree of perceptual and time distortion produced by traditional psychedelic agents. It has effects that most commonly last two to five hours. MDMA is, like LSD, of synthetic origin but not this time by Sandoz. It was first synthesized in 1912 by Merck in Germany, not as a product of interest but as an intermediate chemical in the pathway to developing a drug affecting blood clotting. Some of its basic pharmacological properties were first tested in 1927, on things like blood glucose levels, but its mental effects remained undiscovered. Some further basic experiments were conducted in the 1950s leading to the first published paper describing its chemical properties in 1960. Illicit use began to emerge in the mid-1970s and its psychotropic effects were first described by Alexander Shulgin in 1978.

Following its "rediscovery" in the late 1970s, it wasn't long before MDMA began to be adopted as a drug that could potentially enhance the process of psychotherapy. Its capacity to induce a positive sense of well-being was coupled with engagement in psychotherapy as a way of trying to enhance the development of insight into psychological problems as a pathway to their resolution. By the mid-1980s, MDMA had also become a relatively commonly used illicit drug, known as ecstasy and became particularly popular in dance parties (raves). It was first classified as a restricted schedule 1 substance in the US in 1985.

So, what is the connection of these drugs to the treatment of disorders like depression. To address this, we first need to explore the idea of psychedelic-assisted psychotherapy or psychedelic therapy. These terms generally refer to the combination of ingesting a psychedelic drug whilst engaging in some form of psychological talking therapy. Two variants of this developed in the 1960s. First, the "psycholytic" method involved the use of low drug doses during frequent therapy sessions: drug administration was proposed to enhance the process of psychotherapy, which was otherwise conducted in a relatively normal manner.

"Psychedelic psychotherapy," or the "psychedelic method," was somewhat different. This involved the use of higher doses in relatively few, typically prolonged, therapy sessions to induce more mystical experiences or stronger emotional effects, to try and enable patients to work through challenging mental health problems in a compressed and enhanced manner. This is the treatment I will mostly discuss in this chapter, as it is the approach that is being more systematically developed as a novel treatment approach in the modern day.

Psychedelic psychotherapy typically involves several separate stages. In the first, preparatory stage, the patient undertakes several therapy sessions exploring his or her life history, problems, and customary ways of seeing things. There is a focus on exploring how the patient may emotionally develop through the subsequent treatment as well as providing education as to what the patient may expect in the sessions to come. This is typically followed with between one and three (most commonly two), medication assisted treatment sessions. These are prolonged (all day) and should take place in a quiet, comfortable, and reassuring environment. They usually involve two therapists of opposite sex: this enhances the safety of the environment and therapeutic relationships. The third and final stage of the process is usually referred to as integration. This involves a series of more standard therapy sessions designed to allow the patient to come to terms with their experiences and how these might lead to meaningful change.

What is the evidence that drug enhanced, or psychedelic therapy can be clinically helpful for patients with mental health conditions? Data addressing this question has been sporadically collected since the middle of the 20th century. In fact, the potential therapeutic benefits of psychedelic drugs, especially LSD, were investigated relatively extensively in the 1950s and 1960s, facilitated by Sandoz making the drug available to any psychiatrist who wished to engage in experimental use. Early applications focused on the treatment of schizophrenia and related conditions, but it was progressively recognized that patients with psychotic disorders such as these did very poorly on LSD. However, there was more widespread recognition that individuals with so-called "neurotic disorders" (what we now regard as depression and anxiety) could get significant therapeutic value out of LSD related therapy. Research and clinical programs utilizing LSD were common in the US but also were implemented in the UK and a number of other European countries. In addition to patients with psychosis and neurotic disorders, studies and clinical programs used LSD in a wide variety of groups of patients. This included individuals who would now be diagnosed with personality disorders, patients with addictions and most troubling homosexuals, regarded at the time as "sexual deviants."

A number of studies have been published describing outcomes in relatively large groups of patients treated in centers across both North American and Europe. In 1967 a group from California reported on the outcomes of over 240 patients treated with LSD (augmented in some cases with mescaline, a drug extracted from the peyote cactus which can have powerful hallucination inducing effects) administered in a method relatively similar to that being used in modern day psychedelic assisted psychotherapy.* There was considerable variability in the diagnosis of the patients included in this study, but care was taken to ensure that drug administration occurred in a quiet pleasant setting and the patient was provided with support and companionship (but no active psychotherapy) during the drug treatment itself. A rating of improvement was made by a number of clinicians involved in the care of the patients. 18.9% of patients were rated as being "markedly improved," 26.3% as "substantially improved," and 35.8% as having had "some improvement." 16.9% were "unchanged" and 2.1% reported as worse off than pre-treatment. The greatest benefits seemed to accrue in patients with a psychoneurotic depressive reaction," "immature personality" or an "adjustment reaction."

### LSD and the CIA

Readers with an interest in conspiracy theories may well be interested in a psychedelic treatment controversy that raged in Norway in the early 1990s. A set of beliefs developed in the community that the CIA was funding and leading LSD research in the area of mind control and had control of the supply of the drug through Sandoz. Accusations were made that children were used as 'guinea pigs' in experiments and died as a result and these beliefs attracted at times fairly uncritical national and international media attention. A national truth commission was established in 2001 which ultimately concluded that the claims were unfounded.

* Savage C, Hughes MA and Mogar R (1967) The effectiveness of psychedelic (LSD) therapy: a preliminary report. British Journal of Social Psychiatry 2: 59–66.

It is worthy of note that the CIA was involved in the conduct of extremely dubious LSD experiments but these were mostly conducted during the 1950s, they certainly did not have control over the supply of LSD which Sandoz was distributing freely and it does not make a great deal of sense that they would have specifically restarted this program in Norway in the 1990's rather than anywhere else.

The experiments conducted in the 1950's are really quite shocking. The CIA administered LSD to unknowing prisoners, patients in mental health institutions and other vulnerable individuals. They developed plans to add LSD to the water supply of enemy countries and at one stage planned to order 100 million doses from Sandoz. They even had Eli Lily, a U.S. pharmaceutical company, break the Sandoz patent and work out how to make LSD, so that they had more guaranteed access to a U.S. based supply of the drug.

In 1996, the outcome of LSD treatment in 379 in patients treated in a Norwegian psychiatric hospital, the ominously sounding Modum Bad Nervesanatorium, were reported from treatment that occurred in the years between 1961 to 1976.* Patients were again treated with a range of diagnoses and on average had 5.8 drug treatment sessions. When followed up, 63% of respondents reported that treatment had been helpful with 10% reporting that their symptoms had worsened, at least for some period of time. Treatment of a large group (almost 400) patients during a similar time period was also reported from Denmark with somewhat less optimistic conclusions. Specifically, several adverse events that were considered to be possibly related to treatment including several suicides, attempted suicides, a psychotic reaction, and one homicide were reported. In 1986 the Danish parliament passed a "LSD Damages Law" providing compensation to anyone who had suffered long-term psychological harm from LSD treatment: 151 patients subsequently applied for compensation. It has been argued that the financial incentive to report

* Madsen J and Hoffart A (1996) Psychotherapy with the aid of LSD. Nordic Journal of Psychiatry 50: 477–486.

harm may have elevated these figures and also that the treatment differed quite substantially from what would be reasonable standards of care now, however, this report remains sobering.

The main concern with these early studies of psychedelic use was that they were typically uncontrolled and implemented without the rigor one would now expect in clinical trial research. They do, however, give us a promising sense that psychedelics may be helpful in the treatment of some patients with mental health conditions and this knowledge has persisted, typically outside of the mainstream of psychiatry, since that time. In fact, much of this knowledge was pushed aside, and underground, by the strict anti-drug laws that started to be introduced in the late 1960s. Use of psychedelics, including in indigenous, sacramental, and therapeutic contexts, continued underground over the following decades remaining very much separate from mainstream psychiatry.

Things have changed now, however. We are very much in the middle of a second wave or resurgence of interest in psychedelics, especially in a medical context. And this time, things seem to be happening somewhat differently, certainly with a more modern approach to research and evaluation. The care taken here very much reflects ongoing concerns in the community about these drugs, although even this broader societal context is changing. This was most dramatically seen in a 2020 vote in Oregon to mandate the state government to establish programs to evaluate these drugs and make them available as appropriate. But what has the more recent science unveiled?

The first "modern" evaluation of psychedelic informed psychotherapy that I can find was a report in 2006 of the treatment of nine patients with obsessive compulsive disorder,* not with LSD, however but with psilocybin. Each patient undertook four sessions: in each, they received a differing dose of psilocybin ranging from 25 to 300mg one week apart. They rested with music playing and whilst wearing eyeshades with two "sitters" present in the room to provide support. Psilocybin use was

* Moreno F, et al. (2006) Safety, tolerability, and efficacy of psilocybin in 9 patients with obsessive-compulsive
disorder. Journal of Clinical Psychiatry 67: 1735–1740.

associated with significant short-term alleviation of OCD symptoms, five patients reported "psychologically and spiritually enriching" experiences including the "transcendental" experiences reported by four. However, there were no meaningful differences between the effects of the different doses: even the 25mg dose used as a 'comparator' produced significant benefits, making the results hard to interpret.

Like this study, most modern psychedelic research has moved on from LSD, but not completely. In 2014, a group of Swiss researchers published a small trial involving 12 patients who had significant anxiety associated with a life-threatening illness.* The LSD drug therapy session followed several preparatory psychotherapy sessions and involved the use of a standard LSD dose, or a very low dose proposed to be an active placebo. Participants in the active treatment arm reported a significant reduction in anxiety that persisted for 12 months, and the therapy was not associated with significant side effects. Notably, there were no periods of persistent anxiety, perceptual disturbance, or psychosis. In another recent study, LSD was provided to a group of 12 healthy subjects in a controlled laboratory setting.** This was associated with improvements in positive attitudes and life satisfaction that generally persisted for 12 months and again there were few side effects.

Studies exploring the use of psilocybin assisted psychotherapy over the last decade have been quite diverse: in fact, conducted across a number of clinical groups including patients with treatment resistant depression, cancer-related anxiety and depression, and substance dependence with varying groups of patients ranging from 11 to over 50. In patients with cancer or terminal illness, therapy has generally been associated with improvements in anxiety, and in some cases with reduced depression, with these effects typically persisting during the study follow-up periods, although these have been generally relatively short. Several small studies

* Gasser P, Holstein D, Michel Y, et al: Safety and efficacy of lysergic acid diethylamide-assisted psychotherapy for anxiety associated with life-threatening diseases. J Nerv Ment Dis 2014; 202:513–520
** Schmid Y, Liechti ME: Long-lasting subjective effects of LSD in normal subjects. Psychopharmacology (Berl) 2018; 235:535–545

have also investigated whether psilocybin can enhance the capacity of individuals to quit smoking or reduce excessive alcohol use with promising preliminary results.

What about depression itself? So far, there has been only very limited research exploring the use of psilocybin in patients with depression. In 2016, a group of researchers from the UK published a small "open-label" study (i.e. this study did not involve any form of placebo control) on 12 patients with depression who had failed to respond to at least two different antidepressant medications. Psilocybin was administered during two therapy sessions a week apart and patients also received support before, during, and after each session. Medication dosing was associated with clear psychological effects from about half an hour after the medication was taken to around six hours. There were no major adverse events. The overall level of depression reported by these patients was reduced both one week and three months after medication administration although in quite a number of patients, there was evidence of a significant worsening of their symptoms between the one-week follow-up and when they were seen three months later. In fact, five of the 12 patients were described as having had some form of relapse of their depression by this time.

A second recent study has been published exploring the use of psilocybin in patients with depression, although notably, these were not patients with treatment resistant illness. A total of 27 patients participated in a randomized trial involving the administration of two doses of psilocybin in two separate therapy sessions. 15 patients received treatment immediately and 12 were allocated to a delayed treatment group, having follow-up assessments initially and then treatment some months later. 24 patients completed this study and all assessments. The authors reported a significantly greater reduction in depression in the patients who received treatment immediately, compared to the change in symptoms seen during the waiting period for the second group of patients. The benefits were seen to persist for weeks after the end of treatment but no longer-term follow up or outcomes were reported. Treatment was not associated with serious adverse events, but a headache was common along with patients experiencing challenging emotional and physical sensations such as fear, sadness, and shaking of the body during the drug therapy sessions.

A third study was published in 2021 gathering considerable media attention. This so called "phase 2" study provided either 2 doses of psilocybin, three weeks apart or a daily dose of the antidepressant escitalopram as well as placebos to try and ensure patients did not know what they were receiving. Psilocybin treatment produced a numerical, but not statistically significant, greater improvement in depressive symptoms as well as a significantly greater remission (complete recovery) from depression compared to escitalopram (57% vs 28%). This is certainly promising although it remains unclear whether the patients really remained "blind" (unaware of their treatment group), especially given the strong effects of the psilocybin.

In addition, two recent studies have been conducted investigating the use of ayahuasca with therapeutic intent in patients with some form of depression. Both of these studies included patients who had failed to improve with one antidepressant medication therapy. The first was a small initial investigation with six patients and the second a follow up study by the same research group with a further 17. There was no placebo control in either of these trials. The study was conducted in Brazil and the investigators provided ayahuasca prepared in the local community using what was described as the "standard method." In the first six patients, a substantial and marked improvement in depression scores was noticeable within the first day, the benefit was really quite substantial after a week and persisted a further two weeks later. The effects on thought and sensory perception were short-lived and there were no significant side effects except for vomiting (which was common) and transiently increased blood pressure. A similar pattern was found in the follow up study but neither study reported follow up beyond three weeks post treatment.

Research conducted to date with MDMA has focused on a significantly different clinical group, patients with post-traumatic stress disorder (PTSD). Like depression, PTSD is a disorder that is frequently challenging to treat and often poorly responsive to medication. Patients with PTSD frequently report high levels of depression as well as the core symptoms of PTSD itself. The first study to test MDMA assisted psychotherapy in patients with PTSD was published by US researchers in 2010.* 22 patients received either the real MDMA or a placebo during two drug therapy sessions as well as both preparatory and follow-up psychotherapy. These additional therapy sessions involved two 90 minute sessions before the all-day drug administration, one session the morning immediately after drug administration, and three weekly 90 minute therapy sessions after each drug administration. During the drug administration sessions two therapists provided a therapy that was predominantly nondirective and supportive.

There was a substantial reduction in symptoms of PTSD after each of the two drug administration sessions compared to what was seen in the placebo group. Importantly, PTSD scores remained substantially improved in the patients who had real treatment two months later and these benefits were found to persist over several years in a longer-term follow-up study.** During drug administration, there were some temporary increases in blood pressure, pulse, and body temperature but these were transient. Other potential side effects were also transient and there were no significant adverse events. Unfortunately, this study did not include a systematic assessment of mood or depressive symptoms.

A follow-up study by the same investigators involved the treatment of 26 civil and military ex-service personnel with PTSD.*** Two sessions were again used, one month apart, but on this occasion, participants were randomized to a low, moderate or high dose of MDMA. Clinical

* Mithoefer MC, Wagner MT, Mithoefer AT, et al: The safety and efficacy of +/23,4-methylenedioxymethamphetamine-assisted psychotherapy in subjects with chronic, treatment-resistant posttraumatic stress disorder: the first randomized controlled pilot study. J Psychopharmacol 2011; 25:439–452
** Mithoefer MC, Wagner MT, Mithoefer AT, et al: Durability of improvement in post-traumatic stress disorder symptoms and absence of harmful effects or drug dependency after 3,4-methylenedioxymethamphetamine- assisted psychotherapy: a prospective long-term follow-up study. J Psychopharmacol 2013; 27:28–39
*** Mithoefer MC, Mithoefer AT, Feduccia AA, et al: 3,4-methylenedioxymethamphetamine (MDMA)-assisted psychotherapy for post-traumatic stress disorder in military veterans, firefighters, and police officers: a randomised, double-blind, dose-response, phase 2 clinical trial. Lancet Psychiatry 2018; 5:486–497

outcomes were substantially better in the moderate and high dose group than in the low dose group but there were no differences between the moderate and high dose groups themselves. Several larger more definitive PTSD trials with MDMA have subsequently been commenced but the outcomes of these are not yet available.

The data from these studies suggest that various forms of psychedelic assisted psychotherapy may have value in the treatment of mental health conditions including depression and PTSD. However, clearly this falls into the "more research is needed" camp. The biggest missing piece is knowledge about long-term outcomes. These treatments are often promoted as transformational and potentially curative, often presented in contrast to the need for long-term traditional drug therapy or ongoing psychological treatments. However, at this stage we have really no meaningful information as to whether therapy benefits persist and some of the depression data published to date suggests that relapse rates may be relatively high, as they are with other time constrained treatments such as ECT.

What about safety? Is this something we really should be pursuing given societal concerns about drugs of addiction and abuse? Currently, all of these substances are regulated as restricted or controlled in most countries. However, regulatory restrictions may not necessarily have all that much to do with the safety of various substances that are used by individuals in the community.

In the United Kingdom in 2010, a report was published by the "Independent Scientific Committee on Drugs" (ISCD) addressing this question.* The ISCD was a group of "drug experts" who came together as an independent group to review the overall harms and risks associated with a range of both legal and illicit substances. The harms that were considered include those potentially to the person taking the drug and to others. The expert group scored a wide variety of harms and then ranked all of the considered substances by their overall "harm score." The

---

* Nutt DJ, King LA, Phillips LD; Independent Scientific Committee on Drugs: Drug harms in the UK: a multicriteria decision analysis.
Lancet 2010; 376:1558–1565

highest scoring drugs on this ranking, the most harmful, were alcohol followed by heroin and crack cocaine. Mushrooms/psilocybin were considered to be associated with the lowest risk of harm, LSD was third, and MDMA was fourth lowest. Harms were considerably greater with tobacco and benzodiazepines: the group of drugs including Valium and other common sleeping tablets. The harm scores for psilocybin, LSD, and MDMA were five, seven, and nine respectively compared to 72 for alcohol.

Although it does not completely ameliorate concerns that widespread therapeutic use of these drugs could lead to significant problems of addiction or misuse, there has been no suggestion of this in the limited longer-term trials to date. However, this is certainly something that would need to be carefully monitored should one of these agents become a more common part of clinical practice. Psychiatry has a rather consistent pattern of enthusiastically embracing groups of drugs which turn out to have significant dependence or withdrawal effects—the benzodiazepines and SSRI antidepressants to name two—which become increasingly apparent over time, only really after they enter widespread use.

For now the "psychedelic train" is certainly gaining momentum. A series of companies have been formed in this space to provide commercial, potentially regulated, access to these substances. Others are already setting up clinics, across North America and elsewhere. Research institutes and centers have been established in multiple places to conduct psychedelic research with several receiving large scale donations from Silicon Valley billionaires and prominent authors and podcasters. Legalization of psychedelics in places like Oregon will only add to this momentum. Is this justified? Well, we will just have to wait and see. If, as many proponents seem to believe, these drugs offer a pathway to cure or to more permanently resolve mental illnesses than is seen with existing treatments, they will truly be a god send. Given the limited evidence systematically collected to date, however, we just have to sit back and hope this turns out to be the case.

# 12

# LOOKING FORWARD

So WHAT IS there to have learned from this journey through depression and it's treatment? What are the most useful takeaways for people trying to understand this disorder, recover from it, or trying to help someone else on the pathway to a return to health?

First, I would hope that you would come away with the impression that depression, for better or worse, is not a simple medical problem. It is neither a simplistic disorder of brain chemistry (that is, it is certainly not a disorder of not enough serotonin) nor a weakness in someone's character or will. Depression typically seems to develop as a result of a number of interacting factors in someone's life as well as their genetics and the way they see and perceive the world. Some people are remarkably resilient to the trials and tribulations of day-to-day life, others much less so, but depression seems to have the capacity to rear its ugly head in a wide range of individuals in a wide range of circumstances.

There is no singular explanation and matched to this, no singular solution. Any self-help guru, expert, or well-meaning friend who tells you that you only have to do a specific therapy, meditate, think positive, take a certain drug, eat, or not eat spinach or whatever food or vitamin, and you will be fine, needs to be politely ignored.

I would hope that you would have gained an understanding that the treatment of depression can be straightforward and successful, but it is more commonly complex and challenging. Ideally helping people with depression involves a range of approaches and interventions provided in an integrated and holistic manner. There are very few people with depression for whom treatment will be successful with any one of the approaches described in this book alone.

It is also absolutely crucial to be aware that a biological treatment, a drug, TMS, ECT, or something else, may work extremely well and produce a complete resolution of the symptoms of depression. However, this will not necessarily change what made the person vulnerable to developing depression in the first place. The medication will not give the person a sense of efficacy: that they have overcome their illness, and developed understanding and resilience. Treatment with a biological agent alone will not take somebody anywhere on the journey of their life. Don't get me wrong, depression is a terrible thing and one for which everybody should be able to seek resolution as quickly as possible. However, the development of depression for the first time also has the potential to be a powerful inflection point in someone's life.

There will invariably be something that can be learned from this experience. It might be as simple as "alcohol is not good for me" or "I need to get out of this dead-end job." However, it may be much more complex. Someone might come to understand the impact of traumas that they have experienced during their life, and how these traumas have shaped their characteristics, habits, and coping strategies. These may be challenging to change but finding that they have a role can be an important and crucial first step. Something that can start someone on the pathway to a truly meaningful transformation.

None of this is possible unless you are supported by people who adopt a relatively holistic and integrated approach to the treatment of depression. The physical interventions may be critical but there will always be important psychological dimensions, let alone physical health, lifestyle, and the impact of broader social factors, relationships, and supports to consider.

Another element of the complexity of the treatment of depression that we have explored at length in this book is the inconsistent nature of the responses achieved with most of the accepted and establish treatments for this disorder, especially antidepressant medications, and the side effects that can arise from these therapies. These medications are far from the magic bullets we would like to hope they could be, although for some people, in some episodes of depression, they can make an enormous difference. I think sometimes how medications are prescribed is as much of a problem as the medications themselves. Patients who are repeatedly prescribed medications that are similar to one another, for example, repeated scripts of different SSRIs, when these are not working, are really not getting even vaguely adequate treatment. If medications are not working after several tries, a significantly different approach is warranted. At a minimum, this should involve a reconsideration of the diagnosis and overall management plan. It might involve a decision to try medications from significantly different groups, it may include other physical therapies such as rTMS or a reconsideration of the role of, and approach taken with psychotherapy.

Navigating this process may be challenging for individuals with depression who by the nature of their illness are likely to lack confidence, motivation, and the hope to push on with treatment. It might take the efforts of those around them to assist in this process and to provide a buffer against the sense of failure and self-blame that can arise if they have not been a "good patient" and responded well to initial therapy. Simplistic messages that "depression is treatable," used to encourage people to come forward and seek help when well, can backfire on individuals who do not feel they are following the path expected of them.

This support is a helpful role that you can play in supporting someone along this pathway. I will often encourage patients and their carers to "set the bar high." The overall aim of the treatment of depression is not a simple lessening of symptoms but true recovery. Recovery is a fairly loaded term in the mental health field and has a variety of different meanings. Possibly the easiest way to understand this is as this distinction between two types of recovery. The first—what I will call *clinical recovery*—refers to the idea that a person no longer has any clinical symptoms, that their depression has resolved. This is obviously something that anyone with depression would want to aim for and an admirable goal. The second concept of recovery refers to a process through which a person is able to create and live a meaningful life, whether or not they continue to experience ongoing mental health related symptoms. The definition of meaningful is personal and individual. The person chooses to live in a manner that is in keeping with their personality, values, and desires.

These two forms of recovery are clearly compatible with one another but the second is at least partially determined by how you try and achieve the first. This broader sense of recovery involves the development of a sense of independence, self-esteem, and control over the present and future. This is not going to be helped by clinicians, or well-meaning others, telling someone what to do, or making decisions for them. It will be assisted by care that tries to respect individuality: trying to understand the unique qualities of the individual and how these can be supported to aid them in the process. It will involve the person feeling involved in their care at all levels. From setting the goals to making simple day to day decisions. Decision making involves the requirement for information and education. Not all patients will want the level of information about the options available to them that is contained in this book, but they all deserve to be able to have it if they so desire.

So, what did I mean by "setting the bar high?" I meant having an expectation of achieving so called clinical recovery but ensuring that you respect the principles of true recovery along the way. Patients should have an expectation that with proper treatment, care, and time that their depression will go away. This is not an unrealistic expectation. However, there is, unfortunately, a group of patients in whom this will not be the case. A very small group of patients will have persistent symptoms of depression for a sustained period of time. Another group of patients may well achieve almost complete resolution of symptoms but continue to be troubled by side effects of the medication required to get them there or persistent anxiety, something that can linger after depression resolves. Others will find that the depression goes away but issues from their past, perhaps associated with previous traumas, will have come more to the forefront and continue to impact their quality of life.

Care needs to be taken to respect both of these principles, to push "hard" to get a full resolution of symptoms while supporting an individual on the overall journey to recovery. In regard to the former, patients and their supporters often need to push this agenda, especially with treating doctors. I have mentioned several times the problem of the repeated unsuccessful prescription of medications that are too alike to expect a better outcome. A second common problem is with the timing of treatment changes. If a medication is not working, this will be apparent in weeks and does not require months and months. If there is no change at all after three or four weeks, a decision needs to be made: a higher dose might make sense, or trying something else altogether. If the dose is increased, the response to this should be actively reviewed after no longer than a similar three to four week period, if not sooner.

The situation is a little more complex if there are signs of improvement, even if these are slow. My practice generally is to leave well enough alone under these circumstances. I think you are more likely to do harm than good by pushing doses up when someone is improving, than if you are waiting and watching cautiously.

Similar considerations apply to the process of monitoring and evaluating ongoing psychological treatments. Patients should be encouraged and supported to actively plan with their therapist the form, process, and expected outcomes of therapy. All too often I hear stories of patients who are seeing someone who talks to them about their day-to-day life but is not really engaging in a form of evidence-based psychotherapy that we could expect may make a meaningful difference to their depression itself. This type of support might be valuable and appropriate alongside another form of treatment, such as medication, but often patients have an expectation that they are engaging in therapy that may actually make a meaningful difference to their underlying symptoms and this may not be the case. The type of therapy, its expected outcomes, risks, complications, and especially alternatives, should all be openly discussed with a patient prior to commencement, just as one should do when prescribing a new medication.

Just because a patient is being seen by a CBT therapist does not necessarily mean that CBT might be the right thing, right now. The choice of therapy, the reasons for the proposed choice, and a sensible discussion of alternatives should be undertaken prior to commencement. Referral to a colleague for a more appropriate approach, or the selection of a form of therapy by the patient based on the provision of full and balanced information, should be a routine part of care. In fact, if a therapist only offers one type of approach, for example, CBT, and is not at least occasionally referring patients out for other types of treatment, I think they would need to take a serious look at whether they are really providing informed care and supporting patient choice.

Just as one type of therapy is not going to suit all patients with depression, neither will one type of therapy be suitable all the time in one individual patient. For example, CBT may well be the most useful approach whilst somebody is struggling to get better, but as they recover and are interested in staying well in the longer term, a shift towards a more mindfulness-based approach, or perhaps an approach addressing problematic patterns of long-term relationships could be appropriate. It is the responsibility of the treating clinician to recognize the necessity of these transitions and provide appropriate information and support. However, it is worthwhile for patients and their support people to develop an awareness of this as well as to help their capacity drive the selection of treatment modalities.

Although much of this book has involved a critique of the current methods of managing depression, I also hope that my message is one of optimism. The treatments that we have available right now are reasonable, but I would say, not yet good enough. However, as I have hoped to portray, I do not think that the management of patients with depression in five or 10 years is going to look the same as it does now. There are lots of exciting new treatments becoming available or in development. Not everything that is being tested currently will prove to be useful, or potentially even safe. However, I think it is reasonable to assume that at least some of these treatments will progressively become part of the treatment landscape for patients with depression and this is definitely a good thing.

Having a greater range of treatment choices is not an end in itself but is desirable because it will maximize the likelihood that there will be a treatment option that suits all patients, at all times in their life. We need to have extremely safe, low-cost, and convenient treatment options for patients who first present with depression. These need to be widely available and able to be accessed in a way that minimizes the impact on people's lives. Cheap, safe, and "easy to take" treatment will provide an extremely powerful carrot to ensure as many patients as possible come forward and get treated as early as they can. It is also critically important that new therapies are developed for this phase of depression and are tested and evaluated for safety in children and adolescents.

This might seem blatantly obvious, especially if you are aware that a great proportion of patients who develop depression do so for the first time well before the age of 20. However, it is infrequently, if ever, the case. New treatments are typically evaluated in adult patients and only tested later in younger people, if ever at all. The treatment of depression in childhood and adolescent patients often involves using treatments that have never been tested in people in these age groups. They are used because they work in adults and therefore are assumed to work for younger patients. Or because there are so few treatments that have actually been established to work for those below the age of 18 at all.

We need to do much better than this. Treatments need to be specifically developed and tested in young people thinking about the uniqueness of the adolescent brain, its chemistry, and stage of development.

We should also be more ambitious: it seems possible to develop a treatment for depression in a 15-year-old that when it works means that the depression won't repeatedly recur later in life. This certainly is not the case with standard antidepressant drugs. If anything, people such as Robert Whitaker, author of the provocative book *Mad in America*, have argued that using these drugs increases the likelihood of further episodes in the future. I am not convinced that we really know whether this is true or not but we certainly don't have treatments that can be prescribed with any confidence that they will make a positive difference to somebody's likelihood of developing depression in the decades to come.

Beyond considerations of age group, we also need to increasingly be thinking about the development of treatments based on the stage of illness. Current medication management for depression is "one stage fits all." You take the same drug to get better that you take to try and stay well. I can imagine a time when the choice of initial therapy may be deliberately very different from that required to consolidate and complete recovery and different again from the maintenance strategies used to stay well. Drugs like ketamine and the drugs that are following its development appear to be able to work very quickly, to kick-start the process of recovery, but may be problematic with long-term, or even medium-term use. If *Spravato* is any indication, they may be too expensive for routine longer-term use as well. It may prove sensible to use a drug like this to try to initiate a rapid antidepressant response whilst waiting for a slower acting treatment, be it with medication or something like TMS, to start to work. There then might be another transition as somebody recovers and the focus turns to long-term stability. Psychotherapy might come into its own here although we might also be looking at forms of brain stimulation, such as tDCS or tACS, that a patient could intermittently apply themselves in their own home with few if any side effects.

The critical illness stage that has been a focus of a lot of this book has been the management of patients who have failed to respond adequately to initial forms of treatment. As we have discussed, this is a much too frequent problem. It is, however, one that has become increasingly a focus of attention, especially in the development of new therapies. This focus is clearly very welcome. As it currently stands, research has established TMS as a safe and very effective treatment for this group of patients and it certainly looks like some form of ketamine is likely to be useful. The discovery of the benefits of both of these has spurred major efforts to develop additional treatments. Success with TMS has clearly played a major role in encouraging the entire field of brain stimulation. The breadth of new brain stimulation treatments that have been tested or are being developed now is actually quite impressive.

Not all of these will work. In fact, several companies developing new forms of brain stimulation have gone out of business in the last couple of years as the devices they were developing failed to show the hoped for benefit in clinical trials. This is clearly disappointing for all involved, although it is inevitable. Not all good ideas will turn out to be right. If we take any lessons from the drug development area, we should expect vastly more failures than successes. The chance of a newly developed drug getting through all levels of clinical testing to be released for use in the clinic is usually estimated at about one in twenty. I am hopeful that the hit rate with forms of brain stimulation will be better than this, but there will be lots of failures along the way. It is therefore essential that there is a substantial ecosystem to encourage the development of new ideas, and the testing of these, to maximize the chances that we find new treatments of value.

The discovery of the value of ketamine has also had a substantial catalytic effect. New drug discovery efforts for mental health conditions including depression have really waned in recent decades. There are lots of antidepressant drugs on the market—although as we have talked about, they are not all that good. Many are now off patent and relatively cheap. This is actually a disincentive for companies to invest the money required now to develop a new drug. It takes at least $1 billion to develop a new drug from inception to clinical use. Having to place a new drug into competition with a range of inexpensive off patent generic medications is financially off putting. Companies had also just run out of ideas. Many drugs were made to mimic the original serotonin focused medications but little that is new was coming through.

As ketamine has been recognized as having antidepressant effects, and unusually rapidly acting ones, this has stimulated considerable interest in developing new medications that might act in a similar way, and have the same benefits but potentially fewer problematic side effects. A number of pharmaceutical companies are developing drugs to target the same brain processes as ketamine. Others, like the laughing gas nitrous oxide, are being evaluated by academic clinicians. Some of these options are already being tested in patients, so hopefully, over the next few years, we will see some success coming out of these endeavors.

Of note, the advancement of novel treatment options for patients who struggle to respond well to standard modalities has only been patchily accompanied or supported by the development of new clinical services. The provision of treatment with TMS is leading to a significant change in this. TMS, especially when provided as it should be, as an outpatient, requires the establishment of clinical services that are not insignificantly different from the standard outpatient clinics that have been the mainstay of non-hospital mental health treatment for decades. The development of a range of TMS clinics is morphing in many places into the growth of new services providing an increasing range of "interventional therapies" including ketamine. There is also considerable international interest, and investment in, establishing clinical services for the provision of various forms of psychedelic assisted psychotherapy, which really cannot be adequately provided in a standard consulting room environment. The more that these novel services develop, the more flexibility and capacity will exist for the timely provision of the new treatments that arise in the coming years, let alone the investment environment and availability of financial resources to support new service development. These financial and practical issues seem of less importance than the clinical ones that we have been discussing, but are critical to ensure that treatments can be accessed by the widest range of patients.

# FINAL THOUGHTS

S o HOW DO we wrap this all up? Clearly there is no simplistic model, flowchart, or list of treatments that can encompass all that we have discussed and all that should be taken into account in addressing the treatment and recovery of somebody who is suffering from depression. Diagnosis is important, but equally as important is the emphasis treating clinicians need to place in understanding the uniqueness of each patient with this condition and how its treatment should be guided by this individual understanding. In fact, the treatment of no two patients with depression should or will look exactly alike.

In the following, I will provide some general guidance, in part to summarize much of what I have said already, and in part to provide an accessible summary of practical recommendations. Much of this will not apply to many, although the relevance of some of the treatments may change meaningfully over time. What is not helpful now may well prove to be so down the line. I hope this is useful!

## 1. SEEK HELP FOR DEPRESSION SYMPTOMS

The first port of call on the journey to recovery is to receive an assessment and diagnosis, so start with your family doctor. There are primary care doctors who provide amazing care to millions of patients with depression every year around the world. However, unfortunately, some family doctors are not nearly as up-to-date or expert in the assessment and management of mental health conditions as they should be. If you are not satisfied with the assessment that you initially receive, do not settle for this: seek another opinion.

Please note that this is going to be a journey: the more you can learn about this problem and its treatment the better. Presumably, if you have read this book, you now know more about depression than the vast majority of people, including many clinicians you may encounter. If you are just reading this summary, go back to Chapter 1 and start your education. Alternatively, there are a myriad of valuable resources on the Internet providing information about the diagnosis and treatment of depression. However, make sure you look carefully into the source of the information you receive. There are a number of organizations out there deliberately providing misleading information about mental health conditions, so please beware.

## 2. UNDERGO AN ASSESSMENT

Whether you are being assessed by a family doctor, a specialist psychiatrist, or a psychologist, be prepared to provide detailed information in a variety of the areas that we discussed back in Chapter 1.

Specifically, a thorough assessment is going to involve some exploration of most, if not all, of the following areas:

- The symptoms you are currently experiencing, when they began and how they have evolved
- Any symptoms of mental health problems you have experienced in the past
- Whether family members have suffered depression or other mental health problems
- Your alcohol use and consumption of prescribed and illicit drugs
- Your medical history and any medication that you are taking
- Your background: what life was like for you growing up, what sort of child were you, what were your teenage years like, what sort of stressors and challenging experiences have you experienced during your life and how did you cope with or overcome these?
- What is your family like, what are your important relationships, and what supports do you have?

- What is your lifestyle like, what type of work do you do, what is your diet like, how much do you exercise, what for you are meaningful activities (and how have these all been impacted by your symptoms)?

In addition to these, an assessment of someone with depression will involve an assessment of whether or not the depression is putting the individual at some form of risk. We most commonly think of this in regard to the development of suicidal thoughts but an assessment for depression may also extend to thinking about whether or not the illness results in any degree of risk to others. So do not be surprised to be asked about these things. The person talking to you will most likely enquire as to whether you are feeling hopeless about the future, whether you have thoughts that life is not worth living and whether these thoughts have led you to more detailed thinking about ending your life. Being as open as possible in these discussions, although it may be very hard. It is in your long-term best interests and may provide you with a considerable degree of immediate relief. Many patients find that talking about difficult thoughts like this for the first time actually helps.

## 3. NEGOTIATING TREATMENT

I have used the word "negotiating" here quite deliberately as I would hope for the vast majority of patients that decisions around treatment would be discussed and decided on in a collaborative manner. As we have discussed, the pathway to recovery involves an engagement in decision-making and taking considerable ownership of the treatment that you receive. If you don't feel that you have been provided enough information about the treatment proposed, you have every right to ask questions until you do. If this is a struggle, do not hesitate to make a follow-up appointment. You may want to flag in advance that you require a longer appointment than normal and bring somebody with you as support.

## 4. COMMENCING TREATMENT

As we described in earlier chapters, the initial treatment that you receive for depression will be determined by a range of factors including:

- The severity of your illness
- Whether you have other coexisting mental health or physical health problems
- How much influence social and relationship factors have on your presentation
- How much of the role past traumas are having in the development of your depression now
- The resources and treatments practically accessible to you
- Your preferences and choice

Initial treatment is likely to involve some combination of the following:

- Psychotherapy: most commonly cognitive behavioral therapy
- Antidepressant medication: most commonly a SSRI
- Advice and recommendations around exercise, diet, sleep, and general well-being

## 5. MONITORING OUTCOMES

Once you commence treatment, your progress needs to be regularly monitored by your treating team. Everyone will be hoping that you progressively improve but this is not always the case and if you experience a worsening of your depression, and especially if you start to feel hopeless or notice the emergence of suicidal thoughts, you really should seek out an earlier review. You should ask the people treating you what their expectations are for when you should notice an improvement and use this to guide a schedule of regular review. If you have commenced a new medication and this is not working in four, or at most six weeks, this should be reviewed, and a decision actively made as to whether the dose needs to be increased or the medication changed.

Although depression is usually monitored relatively informally—through the reports of the patient in regard to the severity of their symptoms—some doctors and psychologists will use structured questionnaires to assess the severity of symptoms. Although these are not 100% accurate, they can certainly detect changes in symptom severity that patients may not always notice and can be a really helpful adjunct. In addition, there are a variety of apps that you can download that allow you to monitor your own mood on a daily or weekly basis and these can certainly be useful in staying in touch with how you are feeling and how this is changing over time.

## 6. POST-RECOVERY

When patients recover from depression, there is an extraordinarily strong temptation to want to move on extremely quickly: to get on with their life and as much as possible to pretend it never happened in the first place. Although this is understandable, in the long-term, it will often prove to be unhelpful. What you really want to be doing at this stage is everything you can to ensure that your depression stays away for as long as possible or as some patients can fortunately find, forever.

This may not necessarily be just continuing to do what got you better in the first place. Most psychiatrists will recommend continuing with medication for somewhere between six months and two years after the first episode of depression. The period of time after you have recovered from an episode of depression is the time at which you are most at risk of your symptoms coming back. Therefore, it does make sense to continue with medication for some time but there is far less convincing evidence that medication will keep you well in the long-term.

There are, fortunately, lots of other things you can do to try to maximize the likelihood that you are going to stay well for as long as possible. Things that are just good for your mental health, and often good for your health in general. Some of these are fairly obvious and are activities and changes that it would be wise to be doing anyway. Regular exercise, eating a healthy diet, and limiting your alcohol and drug consumption.

There are others that are also likely to help but may be more challenging. Changing or getting out of dysfunctional relationships, finding more satisfying or meaningful employment (or even finding a job at all), connecting more socially, or engaging in a wider range of meaningful day-to-day or week-to-week activities. Some of these things you can tackle on your own but there will be somewhere seeking assistance from others can be helpful. This could range from a dietician to a social worker or even a personal trainer as well as the sorts of professionals, like psychologists, that you might be already seeing.

Mindfulness, especially mindfulness-based cognitive therapy, falls into this camp as well, as we discussed in Chapter 4. There is good evidence of the role that this can play in preventing depressive relapse and I suspect that even if individuals are not involved in formal mindfulness-based CBT, they are likely to benefit from the regular commitment to a mindfulness based practice anyway.

Then there are those things that are fundamentally more challenging. These have to do with your innate ways of seeing the world, your coping skills, and dysfunctional patterns of behavior that can have arisen in response to your early life relationships, and to losses and traumas throughout your life. These patterns and tendencies often interact with life events to trigger illness recurrence. An event or experience may not be that dramatic but if it particularly coincides with a vulnerability of yours, it may trigger a relapse.

Addressing these issues is in the realm of psychotherapy and personal transformation. There are multiple pathways here to follow. The mainstream approach is to address these with forms of psychotherapy that tackle more fundamental characteristics than might be the focus in the type of CBT or IPT that is often undertaken when somebody is quite depressed. There are multiple forms of psychotherapy that different practitioners would recommend under these circumstances depending on your individual challenges. These could range from variations of traditional psychodynamic psychotherapy to things like DBT or schema therapy (as discussed more in Chapter 4). This is an area where it is very much worth "shopping around." It is worth talking to different therapists, and your doctor, and doing some research online. What you enter into is likely to be a substantial commitment and you will want to go into it with your eyes open.

The last thing to mention here is to think about developing a plan to detect the early signs of emerging relapse. This is often neglected but can be extremely helpful. The idea is that you want to put in place a process for the circumstances when you are starting to slide down the slippery slope back into depression.

This may seem simple. You might think that there is no way you would miss it. And you would certainly want to jump on it early. However, my experience tells me that this is often overly optimistic. The onset of symptoms can be very slow and insidious. People think they are having a bad day, then a bad week, perhaps a bad month. By the time they realize something is seriously wrong, they are well and truly back in a challenging state.

So what to do instead? I suggest that it is well worth your time developing a plan to try and anticipate what you would do should you think you are starting to become depressed again. The first, and most crucial part of this, is thinking about how you would identify the return of depression. Often the most reliable indicator is to think about how you felt early on when you were developing depression for the first time. Can you recall what happened first? Often people experience things like a disruption of their sleep or becoming more anxious before they really start to experience the full-blown symptoms of depression. If this is the case and you can identify these, write them down. As best you can, describe what you can recall it felt like or what changed in what you were willing to do day-to-day.

Second, you need to think about who is going to be the most reliable person to pick up these early signs. It could be you but try and be as brutally honest with yourself as you can. Realistically, will you truly think something is wrong or are you likely to be someone who will downplay it or hope for the best? Don't hesitate to involve someone who cares for you in this plan. Let them know what you think the early signs are and importantly what they should do if they are noticing that you are going down the path.

This is the third part of the plan: what do you do when you detect these signs? This is also worth writing down so there is no confusion at the time. Make it crystal clear: I will go and see my doctor; I will make an early appointment with my psychologist et cetera. You might add in the changes you will make until the appointment. For example, you will exercise for 40 minutes and meditate for 30 minutes every day until you feel back to 100%. If necessary, rope in your loved ones or friends and give them the details of the person you would want to see so that they can follow up and make an appointment for you. This might seem a little bit excessive or dramatic but if you can avert the development of a full-blown depressive illness, you have probably saved yourself weeks, if not months of suffering and this is certainly worth some time and effort.

## 7. WHAT IF YOU ARE NOT GETTING BETTER?

Well, this has really been the focus of most of the book. What I have said can be summarized as concisely as the following:

- **Do not be satisfied if you are on a treatment, and you are not getting better.** Seek review and change if it is required.

- **A review of treatment that is not working should probably include questioning the original diagnosis and considering whether there are other factors.** This includes alcohol, medical illnesses, or psychosocial factors which are undermining the likelihood of progress.

- **Reevaluate dosage.** Increasing doses of antidepressant medications can occasionally help but for many medications, high doses do not do much more than lower doses.

- **If a medication has been partially effective, adding some form of augmentation or booster strategy will usually be considered.** There are a range of these including a number of antipsychotic medications, lithium, a second antidepressant, or thyroid hormone. These can be helpful but be wary of progressively collecting medications and side effects.

- **Be open to trying alternate therapies.** If a medication is not effective at all, you are better off stopping it and trying something else.

- **The more medications that have been tried, the less likely one is going to work in the future.** If you have tried a number of antidepressant medications unsuccessfully, it is time to start to talk to your treating doctor about non-medication alternatives.

- **rTMS is a well-established treatment that is going to be more likely to work than the third, fourth, or fifth antidepressant drug.** It is safe and if available and affordable is certainly worth considering.

- **Forms of ketamine are increasingly available in some places.** These can be very effective, and quickly so, but the long-term safety is less well-established.

- **ECT is a very effective antidepressant treatment and typically safer than most people expect.** It does have risks and side effects, however, so is best reserved for patients who have failed to respond to a number of other treatments or who are extremely acutely unwell and require a rapid antidepressant response.

In the end, if you follow all of the steps and advice given in this book, I cannot guarantee that you will have a great outcome, that you will achieve full recovery, and that your depression will stay away. I am confident, however, that doing these things will give you a much better chance of achieving your goals than otherwise. Everybody's pathway will prove to be slightly different but there are clearly a number of stops along the way that indicate you are on the right track.

If you are supporting somebody who is struggling with depression, please remember that the care and compassion that you can provide is invaluable. This will not always seem to be the case. Someone in the throes of depression may not experience or be able to express gratitude but your efforts are of more importance than you probably will realize.

If you are just reading this out of interest, you or your loved ones have not been touched by depression, I am grateful that you are taking the effort to learn about this challenging topic. I very much hope that the knowledge that you have developed in reading this book will translate into a degree of sensitivity in the way in which you interact with people with mental health problems that you may encounter in the future. We all need to take responsibility for ensuring individuals struggling with mental health problems do not experience discrimination in social and occupational settings and that through knowledge and understanding we provide the sorts of supportive environments that will aid everybody's mental health.

# ABOUT THE AUTHOR

**Paul B. Fitzgerald, MBBS, MPM, PhD, FRANZCP,** is the Head of the School of Medicine and Psychology at the Australian National University (ANU). He is an academic psychiatrist with an MBBS degree, Masters of Psychological Medicine and Research PhD from Monash University. He has conducted an extensive range of experimental studies and clinical trials, focusing on the development of novel treatment options for patients with depression, schizophrenia, obsessive compulsive disorder, PTSD, autism and Alzheimer's disease with a special interest in repetitive transcranial magnetic stimulation (rTMS). He has had continual competitive grant support for over 20 years and published several books, over 500 journal articles and been cited over 25,000 times. He has established multiple clinical services providing rTMS therapy, founded several device and clinical service companies and in 2021 led a national application to the Australian Federal Department of Health which resulted in Medicare funding ($280 million in the first year) for rTMS therapy for patients with depression. He now leads a highly novel school in the ANU bringing together medicine and psychology to further the development of innovative teaching and research programs.